MAGNETIC RESONANCE WORKBOOK

MAGNETIC RESONANCE WORKBOOK

N. A. Matwiyoff, Ph.D.
Director
Center for Non-Invasive Diagnosis and
Chairman
Department of Cell Biology
The University of New Mexico
Albuquerque, New Mexico

Raven Press   New York

Raven Press, Ltd., 1185 Avenue of the Americas, New York, New York 10036

© 1990 by Raven Press, Ltd., All rights reserved. This book is protected by copyright. No part of it may be reproduced, stored in a retrieval system, or transmitted, in any form or by any means, electronical, mechanical, photocopying, or recording, or otherwise, without the prior written permission of the publisher.

Made in the United States of America

Library of Congress Cataloging-in-Publication Data

Matwiyoff, Nicholas A.
    Magnetic resonance workbook.

    1. Magnetic resonance imaging.   2. Proton magnetic
resonance.   I. Title.   [DNLM: 1. Magnetic Resonance
Imaging—problems.   WN 18 M445m]
RC78.7.N83M37 1989   616.07′548   89-10774
ISBN 0-88167-558-X

The material contained in this volume was submitted as previously unpublished material, except in the instances in which credit has been given to the source from which some of the illustrative material was derived.

Great care has been taken to maintain the accuracy of the information contained in the volume. However, neither Raven Press nor the author can be held responsible for errors or for any consequences arising from the use of the information contained herein.

9   8   7   6   5   4   3   2   1

To Janet and Greg

Preface

This primer introduces the beginner to the basic concepts of proton magnetic resonance imaging (MRI) in medicine using models of the proton and tissue magnetization as ordinary magnets. These models provide direct "visual" answers to questions most frequently asked even by students who have a long clinical experience with MRI and who may have participated in a number of magnetic resonance courses. For example, exactly how is the MR signal generated and how is its frequency used to encode position? What do phase, phase coherence, and phase encoding really mean? How do MR signals "decay" and how does this decay affect contrast and intensity in the image? These questions go directly to the heart of the matter of construction and interpretation of images. The fact that they are asked so frequently by students struggling with the subject reflects the somewhat confused state of MRI education. Over the past 40 years magnetic resonance has developed rapidly as a highly sophisticated analytical and structural tool described by an equally sophisticated but difficult language grounded in the quantum mechanics of nuclear magnetic dipoles. Yet the medical magnetic resonance concepts are presented to beginners very rapidly as a potpourri of quantum mechanics, electricity, and magnetism, and often confusing analogies to everyday experience.

Of course, a complete description of the magnetic properties of small particles like the proton does require a quantum mechanical treatment, which also provides the formalism to understand and to apply the full power of nuclear magnetic resonance techniques to biomedical problems. Yet most novices come to this subject with no background in quantum mechanics and only a vague appreciation of the classical concepts of electricity and magnetism that are so important in magnetic resonance. Classical concepts *can* be used to describe the behavior of large numbers of proton dipoles. These constitute the macroscopic tissue magnetization that is manipulated in creating a proton MR image. Given the problems inherent in the "mixed" approach, I have emphasized the classical or macroscopic model in this introductory work because it is easier to understand and it allows a facile visualization of the interactions and processes taking place in proton MRI.

In Chapters 1 through 3 of the workbook I use simple, familiar, two-dimensional models to introduce the central concepts in electricity, magnetism, and MRI. The reader can demonstrate for himself many of these models using two bar magnets, a horseshoe magnet, two compasses (one having the compass needle immersed in a viscous fluid), some iron filings, and a stiff sheet of paper. In Chapters 4 through 6, I extend the treatment to three dimensions where many concepts such as pulse angles and relaxation can be treated more naturally. In Chapter 7, frequency and phase are reconsidered for the purpose of providing more insight into the individual steps of the process of image construction. The reader who does not feel comfortable with the incomplete discussion of phase in Chapter 2 might profit by proceeding directly from Chapter 2 to a preview of Chapter 4 and then Chapter 7, before continuing on to Chapter 3.

I have tried to minimize calculations and the use of equations. Nonetheless, a meaningful discussion of the origin of the variation in signal intensity and contrast encountered with the use of pulse sequences having mixed T_1 and T_2 attentuation (weighting) requires a consideration of the different forms of the exponential time dependence of the signal on the spin–spin relaxation time (T_2) and of equilibrium z magnetization on the spin–lattice relaxation time (T_1). Consequently, I "bit the bullet" and included an explicit discussion of these exponential processes in Chapter 5 and a number of closely related calculations in Chapter 6 to illustrate key aspects of the variation of signal intensity and contrast. I hope the reader will be encouraged to "bite the bullet" as well and read those sections carefully. Doing so will pay big dividends in understanding.

This introductory text is not comprehensive. It is designed as a primer on basic concepts in spin echo imaging that might be a useful companion to the physician or technologist taking one of the many MRI short courses now available. On a more permanent basis, it is intended also as a reference to facilitate the reading of the many clinically oriented reviews, references, and compendia that are being published with increasing frequency.

N. A. Matwiyoff, Ph.D

Acknowledgments

I am indebted to my colleagues M. S. Brown, Ph.D., E. Fukushima, Ph.D., R. Griffey, Ph.D., and C. Haas, M.D., who read the text and provided valuable suggestions and critical comments.

I am especially grateful to Michael Brant-Zawadzki, M.D., for his advice. Without it, this text would not have been written. He was most helpful in the development of Chapters 1 through 3 offering encouragement and suggestions on improving the clarity and simplicity of the text and figures.

I am deeply grateful to my wife Janet for her support and for all her help, not only in preparing this text, but also in her many collaborating efforts in MR education.

N. A. Matwiyoff, Ph.D.

Contents

1 Rudiments of Proton Magnetic Resonance Imaging   *1*

   1.1   What is a proton magnetic resonance image? *1*

   1.2   All substances interact with strong magnetic fields: Very strong interactions can occur for electrical currents and iron bars *3*

   1.3   The interaction of the spinning proton with magnetic fields is weak and the resulting magnetization of tissues containing protons is rapidly established *4*

   1.4   The slight net magnetization of tissue protons in a strong static magnetic field must be detected with a second weaker perturbing field which is imposed at right angles to the static field and which sets the proton magnetization in oscillation *6*

   1.5   The oscillation (resonance) frequency of the proton is a characteristic property that depends on the strength of the static magnetic field that orients it *7*

   1.6   Oscillating fields and currents: The concept of resonance and a simple model for nuclear magnetic resonance *8*

   1.7   Proton magnetic dipoles subjected to an orienting (static) field can be caused to resonate by applying an oscillating magnetic field at the resonance frequency *10*

   1.8   Proton magnetic dipoles oriented in a static magnetic field whose strength is a linear function of position exhibit oscillation frequencies that are linear functions of position: Proton resonance frequencies can encode position *11*

   Summary   The initial stages of proton magnetic resonance imaging (slice selection) *12*

2 Mapping Proton Density in the XY Plane: The Use of Both Frequency and Phase in Proton Magnetic Resonance Imaging   *15*

   2.1   Frequency: Some quantitative considerations *15*

   2.2   The frequency of oscillation of magnetic dipoles can be monitored by the alternating current (voltage) it induces in a coil of wire: More quantitative concepts in electricity and magnetism *17*

   2.3   After selection of the imaging plane with one field gradient an additional magnetic field gradient can frequency encode the position of proton magnetic dipoles along one direction (coordinate) within the plane *19*

xii CONTENTS

2.4 Oscillating magnetic fields and electrical currents: The concept of phase *21*

2.5 Phase encoding of position with a third orthogonal field gradient along the x coordinate *22*

2.6 The central theme of proton magnetic resonance imaging is that the application of three orthogonal field gradients to proton magnetic dipoles in a static (orienting) magnetic field can be used to define the location (x, y, z coordinates) of proton density: The precise order in which the gradients are applied is critical to putting it all together *25*

2.7 Shorthand notation for the processes in proton magnetic resonance imaging: A simplified timing diagram *28*

3 Components of Proton Magnetic Resonance Imaging Systems *31*

3.1 The shape of the fields of some permanent magnets *31*

3.2 Permanent magnets for low-field proton magnetic resonance imaging *33*

3.3 Magnetic fields of wires carrying electrical current *34*

3.4 Resistive electromagnets with an iron core *36*

3.5 Superconducting magnets *37*

3.6 Coils for creating linear gradients in the strength of the static field *39*

3.7 Magnet shimming *40*

3.8 Radiofrequency coils *41*

3.9 Computer requirements *42*

4 The Proton as a Three-dimensional Oscillator *45*

4.1 Introduction *45*

4.2 Concept of spin: Classical *45*

4.3 The magnetization of the sample in three dimensions: Phase revisited *47*

4.4 The B_1 field creates the proton signal: Properties of the oscillating B_1 field *50*

4.5 Creation of the proton signal with an oscillating radiofrequency field: Tilting M away from B_0 and creating phase coherence in the xy plane *52*

4.6 Rotation of magnetization by the B_1 field: Pulse angles *54*

4.7 Free precession of M about B_0 after B_1 is turned off: Only magnetization precessing in the xy plane generates the magnetic resonance signal *56*

5 Repetitive Generation of the Proton Magnetic Resonance Signal in Three Dimensions *59*

5.1 Importance of relaxation processes and initial z magnetization *59*

5.2 Free precession does not last forever: It dies out because of loss of phase coherence: Field inhomogeneities *61*

5.3 Loss of phase coherence owing to the magnetization of the tissue sample itself: Importance of oscillations or fluctuations of the nuclear magnetic moments of water in tissue *64*

CONTENTS xiii

5.4 Loss of phase coherence owing to tissue magnetization: Macromolecules in the water *66*

5.5 The recovery of magnetization along the z axis: General aspects of spin-lattice relaxation *68*

5.6 Spin–lattice and spin–spin relaxation processes are exponential processes characterized by different time dependencies *71*

6 The Influences of T_1 and T_2 on Imaging Time and Image Intensity and Contrast   *75*

6.1 T_1 and the repetition time, T_R *75*

6.2 The use of T_R to increase the difference in signal intensity between tissue structures having different T_1 values: T_1 weighted (attentuated) contrast *77*

6.3 Magnetization in the xy plane lost by field inhomogeneity dephasing can be recovered with a π (180°) pulse: Spin echoes and T_E *79*

6.4 The use of $2T_E$ to increase the difference in signal intensity between tissue structures having different intrinsic T_2 values: T_2 weighted (attenuated) contrast *81*

6.5 Most proton images obtained using spin echo techniques are both T_1 and T_2 weighted (attenuated): A practical consequence is that a reduction in tissue T_1 causes a relative increase in image intensity, but a reduction in tissue intrinsic T_2 causes a relative decrease in image intensity *83*

6.6 Lipid or fat protons contribute to the intensity in proton magnetic resonance images, but not those of the brain *85*

7 Frequency, Phase, and Image Construction Revisited   *87*

8 The Effect of the Repetition Time T_R and the Echo Evolution Time T_E on Contrast in Simple Spin Echo Proton Images of the Head   *97*

9 Review Questions   *105*

Answer Key   *111*

Suggested Reading List   *115*

Subject Index   *117*

1

Rudiments of Proton Magnetic Resonance Imaging

1.1 What is a Proton Magnetic Resonance Image?

The picture shown in Fig. 1-1 is a proton magnetic resonance image (MRI) of a thin (5 mm) slice of a human brain with a resolution in plane of approximately 1 mm × 1 mm. This image of the brain was obtained at depth, noninvasively. The patient was placed in a large, strong magnet, where he acquired a very slight magnetization, so slight, in fact, that even a very sensitive compass could not detect it. The picture elements were then obtained with the aid of an antenna sensitive to the weakly magnetized areas of the patient and converted with a digital computer to an image of the brain recognizable by the eye. After the procedure the patient walked away from the magnet having immediately lost his slight magnetization and having experienced no known deleterious biological effects. The proton MRI bears a strong resemblance to an actual section of a human brain in nearly the same plane taken at autopsy (Fig. 1-2). What is remarkable about the comparison is that Fig. 1-2 is a photograph of the tangible tissue, whereas Fig. 1-1 is actually a graph of the location of the concentration (sometimes called density) of hydrogen atoms (also called protons) that are essential constituents of body water and fat.

The origin of the weak magnetization induced in the body tissue by the strong magnet is the nucleus of the hydrogen atom, which is a small mass of spinning positive charge. Magnetism is associated with the circulation of all charges, positive or negative. A familiar example is the flow of negatively charged electrons (an electrical current) in a wire that is accompanied by a magnetic field surrounding the wire (Diagrams 1-1, 1-2).

2 MAGNETIC RESONANCE WORKBOOK

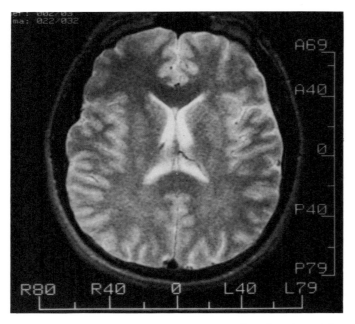

FIG. 1-1. A proton MRI of a human brain taken in axial section: section thickness, 5 mm, in plane resolution 1 mm × 1 mm.

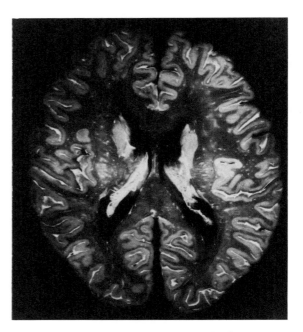

FIG. 1-2. Section of human brain.

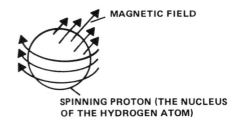

DIAGRAM 1-1. Spinning proton (nucleus of the hydrogen atom).

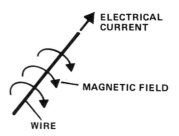

DIAGRAM 1-2. Flow of negatively charged electrons in a wire accompanied by a magnetic field.

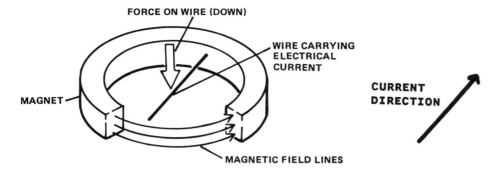

FIG. 1-3. A wire conducting an electrical current in the direction indicated would be pulled down into the center of the static magnetic field.

1.2 All Substances Interact with Strong Magnetic Fields: Very Strong Interactions Can Occur for Electrical Currents and Iron Bars

All substances become magnetized, to a greater or lesser extent, in strong magnetic fields because magnetic fields can cause charges to flow or cause moving charges to align in preferred directions. A familiar example of this force, which is the basis for electric motors and meters, is sketched in Fig. 1-3. The origin of the force is the "push" that magnetic fields exert on moving charges—for the directions of magnetic field and electrical current shown in Fig. 1-3, the magnetic field pulls the current in the same direction it is already traveling, and the wire is attracted into the center of the magnet where the field is greatest. Reversal of the current would result in a magnetic field push against the current and the wire would be repelled from the strong part of the field to reduce the effects of this push.

Another familiar example is the magnetization of a bar of iron in a strong magnetic field, as sketched in Fig. 1-4. When all the domains *that can line up are aligned*, the bar is then completely magnetized at that field strength and will stay that way unless a strong random force, such as heat or mechanical shock, forces the domains out of alignment. When taken out of the field, the bar is a permanent magnet that will attract iron filings or

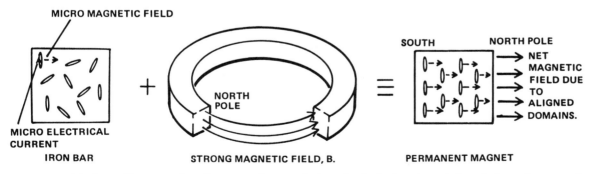

FIG. 1-4. This figure illustrates the alignment of magnetic domains in the iron bar. A domain is a microcrystal in the structure in which there is a net flow of electrons in a closed loop, i.e., the domain represents a microcurrent of electricity and a small magnetic field. The external magnetic field exerts a force on the flowing current, which attempts to align the domain such that its magnetic field is parallel to the external magnetic field. The domains align slowly because they are held tightly in the crystal lattice of the iron bar.

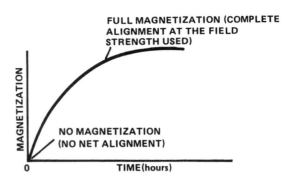

DIAGRAM 1-3. Exponential process required for complete magnetization. Note that *not* all domains necessarily line up, the force of the field being opposed by forces in the iron crystal lattice holding the bar together. To obtain more complete alignment, the magnetic field strength must be increased.

other bar magnets. This is an example of extremely strong magnetic interactions. The time required to achieve complete magnetization at the field strength used is very long (many hours) and follows an exponential process, as shown in Diagram 1-3.

1.3 The Interaction of the Spinning Proton with Magnetic Fields is Weak and the Resulting Magnetization of Tissues Containing Protons is Rapidly Established

In analogy to the forces exerted on current carrying wires and iron bars, strong magnetic fields also exert forces on the protons of tissue, forces that tend to twist the spinning charge of the nucleus so that the weak magnetic field of the spinning charge is parallel to the direction of the strong orienting field (Fig. 1-5). Without the orienting magnetic field, the protons can assume any orientation and there is no net magnetic field associated with the tissue sample. When the tissue is placed in a strong magnetic field (called B_0), the magnetic forces attempt to twist the spinning nuclear charges so that the proton magnetic dipoles are aligned parallel to the orienting field in a low energy state. The forces are weak, however, because the flow of charge (current) associated with the spinning proton is very small. The magnetic forces are opposed by nonmagnetic thermal forces that result in a rapid random movement of the molecules in the lattice of the tissue. These thermal forces cause some of the spinning protons to occupy a higher energy state in which the spinning nuclear charges have their magnetic dipoles antiparallel, or opposed to the B_0 field. The very small excess number of protons in the low energy state relative to the high energy state confers a weak net magnetization M on the tissue sample.

In contrast to the strong magnetism (magnetic forces much stronger than thermal forces) acquired by iron bars in an orienting or static field, the weak magnetization acquired by tissue containing hydrogen in fat and water molecules is acquired quickly. Depending on the tissue type, the time it requires is less than a minute. Nonetheless, an exponential process also characterizes the acquisition of magnetization, as shown in Diagram 1-4. Note that when the tissue is removed from the static magnetic field, it loses magnetization by the same exponential process and becomes de-

RUDIMENTS OF PROTON MRI 5

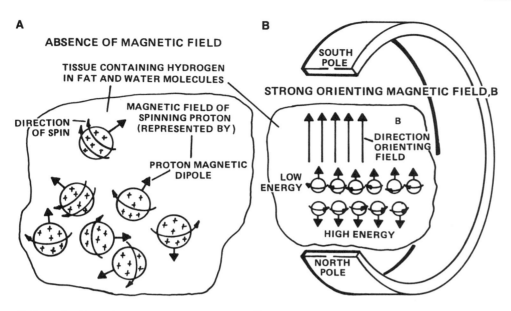

FIG. 1-5. The alignment of spinning protons in a strong orienting static field B_0 and the generation of tissue magnetization M. No preferred orientation of the protons is shown (**A**). The individual magnetic dipoles are randomly oriented and there is no net magnetic field due to the protons. In a strong magnetic field, **B**, the magnetic forces align a few spinning protons, of which more have their magnetic dipoles parallel to the field of direction than anti-parallel (opposed) to the field direction. This confers a weak net magnetization, M, on the tissue, which is depicted in **C**.

magnetized in less than a minute. In this case the thermal forces are much larger than the magnetic forces.

The strength of magnetic fields is measured in Gauss (G) or Tesla (T; 10,000 G = 1 T). As reference points, note that the strength of the average magnetic field of the earth is ~0.5 G or 0.00005 T. The field strength of an iron bar magnet that has undergone magnetization at the highest field strengths might be ~1.0 T at its north or south poles. The range of strengths of the magnets used in *most* proton MRI devices is 0.35 T to 1.5 T. The net magnetization exhibited by tissue protons outside the bore of a 1.5-T magnet is much less than the strength of the earth's magnetic field, or less than 0.001 G.

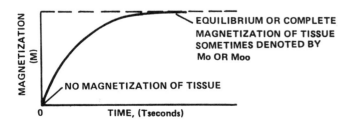

DIAGRAM 1-4. Exponential process in acquisition of magnetization by tissue.

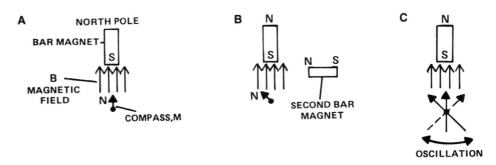
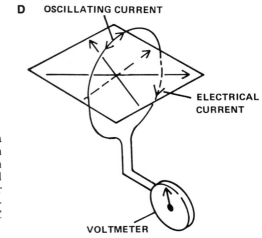

FIG. 1-6. A compass needle oriented in a magnetic field can be set in to oscillation by a second magnetic field. **A:** Orientation of M. **B:** Perturbation of M by a second bar magnet. **C:** Removal of second bar magnet. **D:** Detection of oscillation: an oscillating magnetic field will induce an AC current in a coil.

1.4 The Slight Net Magnetization of Tissue Protons in a Strong Static Magnetic Field Must be Detected with a Second Weaker Perturbing Field Which is Imposed at Right Angles to the Static Field and Which Sets the Proton Magnetization in Oscillation

The net magnetization (M) of tissue protons placed in a 1.5-T field (B_0) corresponds to a weak tissue magnet of strength ~0.001 G or 0.0000001 T. The detection of this weakly induced field in the presence of the much stronger static field would require measurements of nearly impossible precision, greater than 1 part in ten million (10^{+7}), which nonetheless have been the subject of some interesting physics experiments. Another approach to the detection of M, which is at the heart of proton MRI, is to perturb or disturb the net magnetization from its equilibrium alignment with B_0 and then measure the realignment of M with the static field.

A simple easy-to-test model to show how this might be accomplished is sketched in Fig. 1-6. The model consists of a compass representing the M of the proton magnetic dipoles, a strong bar magnet representing the static field B_0, and another bar magnet representing the second perturbing magnetic field.

In A (Fig. 1-6), the magnetization M is oriented along the field lines of a strong bar magnet. In B, a second bar magnet in the same plane as the compass and the first bar magnet is used to deflect M from its alignment, the direction of deflection arising from the repulsion of the two north poles. When the second bar magnet is suddenly removed, the compass will be observed to oscillate about the field direction of the first bar magnet as in C, eventually settling down to its original position. We measure the oscillating return of the magnetization M to its original (equilibrium) position by taking advantage of Faraday's Law: a changing magnetic field can induce a current (voltage) in a loop or coil of wire. For the oscillating M shown in D, an oscillating current (AC) and a voltage will be induced in the coil. This constitutes the magnetic resonance *signal*. As discussed in Section 1.1, the origin of the current is the force that the magnetic field exerts on the electron. Note that the converse is also true—an oscillating current in a coil will also have an associated oscillating magnetic field.

This is a simplified two-dimensional representation of the oscillation of the net proton magnetization, M. By its very construction, a compass needle is forced to oscillate in two dimensions. As we shall see in Chapter 4, the proton magnetization can oscillate in three dimensions, considerably complicating the description of the time dependence of proton magnetization subjected to the combined influence of static and perturbing magnetic fields. For now, we will retain the model of a two-dimensional oscillator for M to simplify the discussion of the elements of proton MRI.

1.5 The Oscillation (Resonance) Frequency of the Proton is a Characteristic Property That Depends on the Strength of the Static Magnetic Field That Orients It

The magnetic force on the spinning charge of a proton is greater at high magnetic fields than it is at low magnetic fields. A consequence of the increased force at high magnetic fields is that more protons occupy the low energy state with their magnetic dipoles aligned with the field. Less obvious is the increase of the oscillation or resonance frequency of the protons with an increase in the strength of the magnetic field. A simple model for the increase in this resonance frequency is depicted in Fig. 1-7.

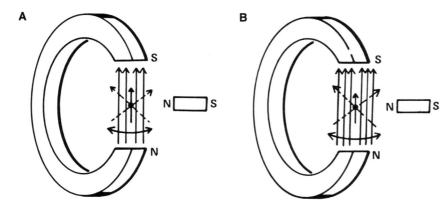

FIG. 1-7. The oscillation frequency of a compass needle originally oriented in a static magnetic field and tipped out of alignment using a second bar magnet (N—S) depends on the strength of the static field. When so perturbed, the compass in the stronger magnetic field of magnet B will oscillate to equilibrium with a higher frequency than an identical compass in the weaker field of A.

In the case of proton magnetic dipoles, there is a linear relationship between the resonance frequency and the strength of the static magnetic field—the resonance frequency for a 1-T static field is twice that for a 0.5-T field. The relationship between the strength of the static magnetic field and the oscillation (resonance) frequency can be expressed by the simple equation:

$$\nu = \text{constant } (\gamma) \times B_0$$

which in various forms is known as the Larmor equation where ν is the Larmor frequency of the proton. The constant, γ, is known as the magnetogyric ratio of the proton. It is a fundamental constant that summarizes the relationship between the strength of the proton magnetic dipole and the momentum associated with the spinning mass of the proton. For bar magnets on a spring, this type of constant would be small for a heavy bar magnet of a given dipole strength and large for a light bar magnet of the same dipole strength—that is, the light bar magnet would have the higher oscillation frequency in the static field. The magnetogyric ratio of the proton is approximately 42,600,000 (actually 42,570,000) cycles/sec per T. One cycle/sec is one Hertz (Hz) and a million Hertz is called a megahertz (MHz). So the magnetogyric ratio of the proton is more conveniently expressed as 42.6 MHz/T.

The oscillation, resonance, or Larmor frequency of the proton in a 0.35-T field is:

$$\nu = 42.6 \text{ MHz/T} \times 0.35 \text{ T} = 14.91 \text{ MHz}$$

The proton resonance frequency in a 1.5-T field is:

$$\nu = 42.6 \times 1.5 = 63.9 \text{ MHz.}$$

These frequencies seem high but as reference points, note that the *electric* fields of FM radio stations oscillate in the 100-MHz range and the frequency of visible light is 100,000,000 MHz.

1.6 Oscillating Fields and Currents: The Concept of Resonance and a Simple Model for Nuclear Magnetic Resonance

We have called the oscillation or Larmor frequency of the proton the *resonance* frequency. Resonance is a familiar concept. When a tuning fork is struck, an identical initially motionless tuning fork will be set in vibration even if it is as far away as 10 meters. The tuning forks are said to be in resonance because their natural frequencies match. Sound waves impinging on the second fork give the fork prongs tiny pushes whose frequencies match the natural frequency of the fork, and consequently each successive push will increase the amplitude of vibration. Another example is pushing someone on a swing—strength is less important than the timing of gentle pushes in rhythm (resonance) with the motion of the swing to achieve high amplitudes of motion. A more obscure example of resonance is the collapse

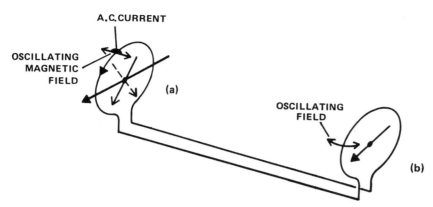

FIG. 1-8. Idealized resonance circuit. This idealized resonance circuit is composed of two identical bar magnets with identical oscillation frequencies. If bar magnet (a) is set into oscillation, it will induce an alternating current in the circuit with an oscillating magnetic field at right angles to the current. What happens at magnet (b) which initially is at rest? The AC will flow through the circuit accompanied by the oscillating field which will be initially at right angles to bar magnet (b) and will exert a resonant torque on it. Very soon bar magnet (b) will be oscillating at the same frequency as bar magnet (a)—it will *be in resonance with (a)*.

of a bridge in England in the early 19th century caused by troops marching in resonance with the natural frequency of the bridge.

Resonance is also common to electromagnetic systems. A simple resonant circuit is sketched and described in Fig. 1-8. It provides a fair model for how we actually observe nuclear magnetic resonance. The strong static magnetic field used in MRI defines the orientation of the magnetic dipoles of the nuclei in our sample. We then place a loop of wire around the sample so that when a short burst of alternating current is passed through the wire, the oscillating magnetic field is at right angles to the oriented nuclear dipoles and sets them into oscillation (the frequency of the oscillating magnetic field must match the resonant frequency of the nuclear dipoles for this to occur). We then turn the AC off, the nuclear dipoles continue to oscillate, and we can detect the oscillation by the voltage induced in the same or another coil, which acts as a receiver antenna.

The matching of the frequencies of the oscillators is a necessary condition for the resonance to occur. For example, in the idealized model of Fig. 1-8, if bar magnet (a) were mounted on a tightly wound spring so that its natural oscillation frequency were high, and bar magnet (b) on a very loosely wound spring so that its natural oscillation frequency were very low, then resonance would not occur because bar magnet (b) could never keep up with the rapid magnetic field oscillations of the wire induced by bar magnet (a). (Check it with a compass immersed in a viscous fluid. Orient the compass south pole with the north of a strong bar magnet. For a slow movement of the bar magnet transverse to the N-S axis of the compass, the compass will oscillate slowly in rhythm. But a rapid movement of the bar magnet back and forth across this axis will result in no movement of the compass.) We change the oscillation frequency of the nuclear magnetic dipoles by increasing or decreasing the static field strength.

1.7 Proton Magnetic Dipoles Subjected to an Orienting (Static) Field Can be Caused to Resonate by Applying an Oscillating Magnetic Field at the Resonance Frequency

A simple, experimentally verifiable physical model of magnetic resonance was introduced in Section 1.6. The application of this model to proton dipoles is sketched in Fig. 1-9. The proton magnetic dipoles are oriented in a static field of strength B_0 and consequently will have a resonance frequency of $v = \gamma \times B_0$. A loop of wire is now introduced into the field and oriented such that when an oscillating current is passed through it, an oscillating field B_1 occurs perpendicular to the orientation of the proton dipoles (perpendicular to B_0). If the frequency of the current is such that B_1 oscillates at v, resonance occurs and the proton dipoles oscillate at their resonance frequency. If the oscillator (B_1) is turned off, the protons continue to oscillate and if a loop of wire attached to a voltmeter is introduced into the field with the same orientation as the oscillator, the oscillating magnetic field of the proton dipoles will induce a voltage. This is the proton magnetic resonance signal.

The oscillator coil is called the *transmitter coil* and the detection coil is called the *receiver coil*. Often the same coil is used for exciting the protons to resonance and receiving the subsequent signal. In that case, the coil is often called a *transceiver*.

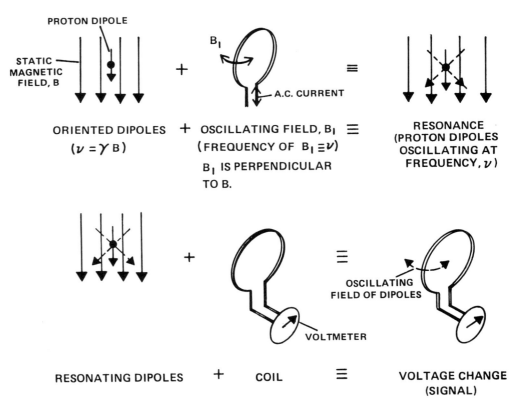

FIG. 1-9. An oscillating B_1 can induce proton dipoles to resonate. The resonating dipoles can induce an AC in a receiver coil.

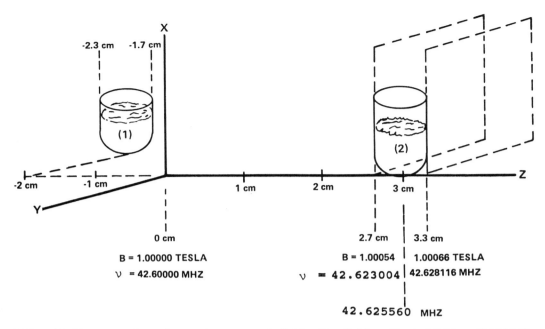

FIG. 1-10. Two test tubes of water in a magnetic field with a field gradient of 2 G/cm (0.0002 T/cm) and a consequent gradient in resonance (Larmor) frequencies.

1.8 Proton Magnetic Dipoles Oriented in a Static Magnetic Field Whose Strength is a Linear Function of Position Exhibit Oscillation Frequencies That are Linear Functions of Position: Proton Resonance Frequencies Can Encode Position

The title statement of this section is central to proton MRI. Known, linear gradients of static magnetic fields can be achieved readily. The following is an example of a linear gradient in the static magnetic field: at 0 cm (the reference point), the field is 1.000000 T; at 1 cm from the reference point, the field is 1.000002 T; 2 cm, 1.000004 T; 3 cm, 1.000006 T; and 4 cm 1.000008 T. If imposed, these gradients create a linear, known gradient in proton oscillation frequencies. If the frequencies can be measured, then the proton resonance frequencies can be used to specify location. In proton imaging, gradients as large as 2 G/cm (or 0.0002 T/cm) are used. This creates a gradient in the proton oscillation frequencies of $0.0002 \times 42.6 = 0.00852$ MHz/cm or 8,520 Hz/cm (or 8.52 KHz/cm).

Suppose we have two 6-mm diameter test tubes of water lined up in a magnetic field of $B_0 = 1$ T (ν of water protons = $\gamma B = 42.6 \times 1 = 42.6$ MHz) and a magnetic field gradient of 0.0002 T/cm in the configuration shown in Fig. 1-10. The center of the magnet is at 0 cm, where the magnetic field is exactly 1.0000 T and the resonance frequency of the protons in the water molecules is 42.60000 MHz. If for some reason, as in an imaging study, we wanted to obtain the proton magnetic resonance of the water protons in test tube #2, which is 3 cm from the center of the magnet, how would we accomplish this? The known gradient in the magnetic field ensures that protons at the low field (1.00054 T) edge of the tube would oscillate at $\nu = 42.623004$ MHz, the water protons at the high field edge would oscillate at 42.628116 MHz, and those at the center of the tube at 42.625560 MHz. To excite or to oscillate all the protons in tube #2, we would require an oscillator that has a central frequency of 42.625560 MHz with a distribution of frequencies of ±0.0025560 MHz about the central frequency. This is the band width of the oscillator (2.556 KHz). As any ham operator knows, construction of an oscillator (transmitter) that has a finite band width (which does not put out a single pure frequency) is relatively straightforward. It is left as an exercise to calculate the frequency and band width of the oscillator required to excite or resonate the protons in tube #1.

Note that with the application of a static field gradient and the use of a transmitter with a finite band width we define the imaging plane shown in Fig. 1-10. All protons in test tube #2 oscillate at the same band of frequencies, as would the protons in all test tubes far off the Z axis, but in the plane sketched. Protons in the other test tube (#1) are not excited because their oscillation frequencies are much lower than the central frequency (plus band width) of the transmitter selected. If, at this stage, we wanted to detect the protons at resonance in tube #2, we could employ a receiver tuned to 42.625560 MHz ± 2.556 KHz.

Summary: The Initial Stages of Proton Magnetic Resonance Imaging (Slice Selection)

The initial stages in proton MRI can be summarized with the aid of Fig. 1-11. The patient is placed within the bore of a strong magnet that has a linear gradient in the static field, B_0. Within a few seconds, the body acquires a slight net magnetization caused by the alignment with B_0 of a slight excess of proton magnetic dipoles in water and fat throughout the body. The alignment of protons in three different planes only is shown in Fig. 1-11. Because the magnet has a linear field gradient in the direction shown, the protons in the plane of the head have a higher oscillation frequency than those in the plane of the abdomen, for example. We can excite

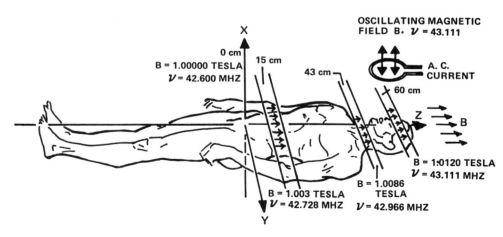

FIG. 1-11. Summary of initial stages of proton MRI.

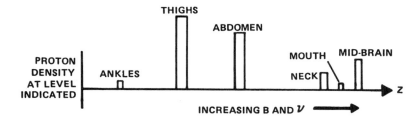

DIAGRAM 1-5. Schematic one-dimensional proton densities in planes throughout the body.

to resonance the protons in the plane of the head by passing a burst of AC current through a coil so that the oscillating magnetic field associated with the current is at right angles to the aligned dipoles and has the frequency of 43.111 MHz. Once the protons have been excited to resonance, they can be detected with a receiver tuned so that a 43.111 MHz oscillating magnetic field will induce a "large" AC current and voltage charge. The magnitude of the current will be proportional to the net magnetization, and hence the number of protons, in the plane excited. Protons in other planes in the body could be excited, and detected, by tuning to other frequencies, e.g., 42.728 Hz for the abdominal plane depicted. With these procedures the most rudimentary of proton images of the body could be constructed—they would consist of graphs of proton concentration (density) in body water and fat as a function of position along the z or long axis of the body. In effect, the method would provide projections of proton density in narrow planes (3 mm–10 mm thick) along the z axis, such as that depicted in Diagram 1-5.

To construct proton MRIs of the type shown in Section 1.1., it is necessary to map the location of proton density not only along the z axis, but also in the xy plane, a subject we will take up in the next chapter. In mapping location in the xy plane, we use both the *frequency* and *phase* of the oscillation (resonance) of proton magnetic dipoles.

QUESTIONS FOR CHAPTER 1

Pick out the one false statement for each of the following:

1. A proton magnetic resonance image is:
   - a graph of the concentration of hydrogen atoms in body water and fat
   - obtained using invasive techniques
   - a map of the weak magnetization induced in body protons by a strong magnet
   - obtained with the aid of antennas (coils) sensitive to the magnetization induced in the body protons

2. Magnetic fields are associated with:
   - spinning charges
   - direct electrical currents
   - gyroscopes
   - alternating electrical currents

3. Magnets:
   - attract ferromagnetic objects
   - exert a force on wires carrying electrical current
   - can "magnetize" all materials, to a greater or lesser extent
   - slowly induce a permanent magnetization in body tissue

Continued on page 14.

QUESTIONS FOR CHAPTER 1 *Continued.*

4. The strength of a static magnetic field:
   —is measured in units of G or T
   —has no effect on the appearance of a proton MRI
   —is linearly related to the proton resonance frequency
   —of a coil can usually be increased by increasing the electrical current flowing through it

5. An oscillating magnetic field:
   —is of little utility in proton MRI
   —can be created by passing an alternating current through a coil
   —is used to tip proton dipoles out of alignment with the strong static magnetic field
   —is associated with proton dipoles returning to alignment with a static magnetic field

6. Resonance:
   —is a concept familiar to experience with tuning forks, electrical circuits, and the buffeting of bridges by winds
   —is a phenomenon unique to proton nuclear dipoles
   —frequencies of proton magnetic dipoles can be increased by increasing the strength of the static magnetic field

7. A proton magnetic resonance signal:
   —contains information about the concentration or density of mobile protons in tissue
   —has a frequency that depends on the strength of the static magnetic field
   —cannot provide information about the spatial location of the proton density

2

Mapping Proton Density in the XY Plane: The Use of Both Frequency and Phase in Proton Magnetic Resonance Imaging

2.1 Frequency: Some Quantitative Considerations

Consider the oscillating magnetic dipole sketched in Fig. 2-1. It might be a bar magnet on a coiled spring set into oscillation by moving the N pole to the $+1$ position and then releasing it, or it might be a proton magnetic dipole in a strong static field along the z axis set into oscillation by a transmitter coil. As the magnetic dipole oscillates from the $+1$ to the 0 to the -1 positions and then back again, the time dependence of the N pole positions will follow the oscillatory pattern depicted. In order to track the time dependence of the motion of the dipole in a standard, compact mathematical form, the projection of the magnitude of the dipole on the x axis as a function of time is actually graphed. The time dependence (t = 0 through f) of the projection of the dipole is sketched in Fig. 2-2.

The motion of the dipole and the magnitude of its projection on the x axis is periodic and describes the cosine function of many periodicities common to our experience, e.g., the motion of pendulums and the transmission of electromagnetic waves by radio transmitters. One cycle of the periodicity in the example of Fig. 2-1 is the oscillation of the dipole from $+1$ through 0 to -1 and then back to the $+1$. As shown in the figure, this definition of one cycle also corresponds to one complete pattern of the time dependence of the projection of the amplitude of the magnitude of the magnetic dipole on the x axis, after which the pattern repeats itself. The frequency of the oscillation is defined as the number of cycles com-

16 MAGNETIC RESONANCE WORKBOOK

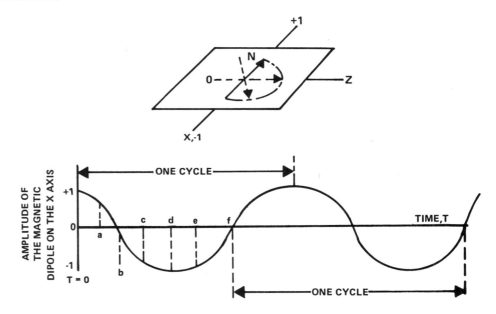

FIG. 2-1. Definition of one cycle of oscillation for the model of the oscillating proton dipole.

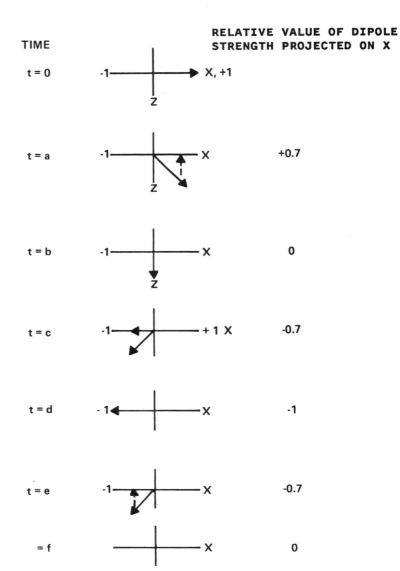

FIG. 2-2. Projections of the value of the strength of the proton dipole on the x axis for the times shown in FIG. 2-1.

pleted in one second. If one cycle is completed per second, the frequency is one cycle/sec or 1 Hz. If one cycle is completed in a msec (0.001 seconds), the frequency is 1/0.001, or 1,000 Hz. If one cycle is completed in a microsecond (μsec; 0.000001 sec), then the frequency is 1/0.000001, or 1,000,000 Hz, or 1 MHz.

2.2 The Frequency of Oscillation of Magnetic Dipoles Can be Monitored by the Alternating Current (Voltage) It Induces in a Coil of Wire: More Quantitative Concepts in Electricity and Magnetism

This subject was discussed in the last chapter. We reemphasize it here with the introduction of some important concepts in electricity and magnetism that have general utility in nuclear magnetic resonance. The force that a uniform magnetic field exerts on moving charges (current-carrying wire) is illustrated in Fig. 2-3A, which also depicts the shape of the magnetic field that results when the circular field of the current-carrying wire interacts with the uniform field. The magnetic field lines reinforce below

A   UNIFORM FIELD + CURRENT CARRYING WIRE = RESULTANT MAGNETIC FIELD

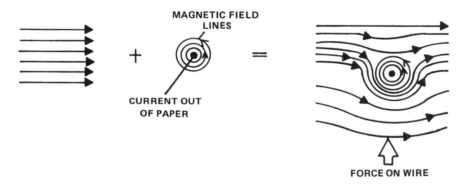

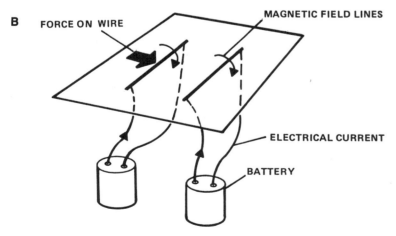

FIG. 2-3. A: Uniform field and current carrying wire-resultant magnetic field. **B:** Direction of the force on adjacent wires carrying electrical current in the same direction. **C:** Oscillating electrical current induced by an oscillating magnetic moment. **D:** Frequency of oscillation and voltage induced by the oscillating magnetic moment in FIG. 2-3C.

FIG. 2-3. *Continued next page.*

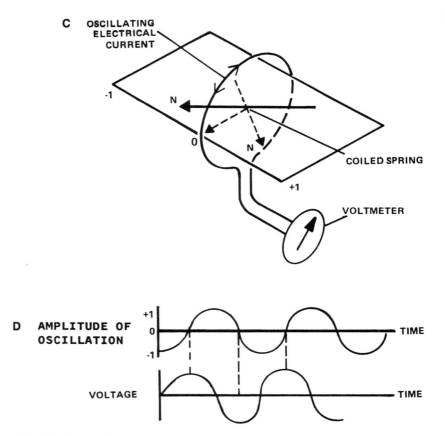

FIG. 2-3. *Continued.*

the wire but interfere above it with a resultant distortion of the original uniform field. The force on the current-carrying wire is directed from the reinforced flux lines to interfering flux lines. The forces can be visualized by the simple experimental arrangement shown in Fig. 2-3B. If one passes electrical current in the same direction through two parallel wires, the wires will move (be forced) closer together; if the current in the two wires moves in different directions (reverse the leads on one battery) then the wires will be forced apart. Empirically, the current, magnetic fields, and forces obey the right hand rule sketched below, which is a coordinate system formed by extending the thumb, forefinger, and middle finger at right angles in the directions indicated in Diagram 2-1.

The fascination and utility in electricity and magnetism is that all the fundamental relations are reciprocal. In the simple example under consideration here, e.g., reciprocity means that if we *force* a wire capable of carrying a current through a magnetic field, then current will flow through it in the direction obeying the right hand rule. The greater the force and the field, the greater the electrical current driven by this *electromotive force* (voltage). Similarly, if we change the magnetic field in which a loop

DIAGRAM 2-1. Relative directions of a magnetic field, the current flowing in a wire, and the force on the wire.

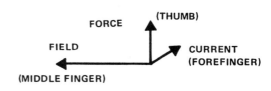

of wire is immersed, then a current will flow through the loop in direct proportion to the rate of change of the magnetic field. This latter aspect of Faraday's Law is responsible for the alternating current induced in a receiver coil by the oscillation of magnetic dipoles. A simple model is shown in Fig. 2-3C. If we twist the spring loaded bar magnet from its rest position at 0 to the -1 position shown, and hold it there, the voltmeter will deflect and return to the original position. If we then release the magnet it will oscillate with a frequency that depends on the tightness of the spring holding it. The maximum current or voltage will be induced in the wire when the maximum number of magnetic field lines pass through the wire the most quickly (Figs. 2-3D). It is as though the force field of the magnet "pushes" the mobile electrons in the wire in a direction that is at right angles to the field and the direction of the force on the oscillating dipole. What we will observe is that the voltmeter will also oscillate:

1. The meter needle will have a maximum deflection when the bar magnet is passing 0 because the greatest density of magnetic field lines run along the N-S axis of the magnet.

2. The direction of deflection of the needle will depend on the direction of oscillation of the magnet, $+1$ to -1 or -1 to $+1$ in accordance with the right hand rule.

Now the principle of reciprocity that we introduced earlier would suggest that *if an oscillating current is passed through a loop of wire, there will be an oscillating magnetic field at right angles to it.* Further, the frequency of the oscillating magnetic field is equal to the frequency of the alternating current.

2.3 After Selection of the Imaging Plane with One Field Gradient an Additional Magnetic Field Gradient Can Frequency Encode the Position of Proton Magnetic Dipoles Along One Direction (Coordinate) Within the Plane

Fig. 2-4 shows an imaging plane of proton dipoles selected and excited in the manner described in Sections 1.7 and 1.8. Initially, all protons are resonating within the same band width, which is defined by the static gradient used and the narrow band selective frequency excitation employed, both of which are now turned off. We can thus precisely define the location of the protons within a relatively narrow plane. How do we locate protons within the plane? By using additional field gradients at right angles to the gradient used to define the plane or slice. We will illustrate in this section how turning a static field gradient along the y direction will change the frequency of oscillation along the y direction across the plane— we can frequency encode position along the y direction.

As a physical model for how this might be done, imagine a compass needle already oscillating in the static field of a bar magnet held far away. What happens when the bar magnet is brought closer and closer? You can verify that the compass needle oscillates more and more quickly. This is caused by an increase of the static field strength and consequent increase of the restoring force on the compass needle. Similarly in our proton mag-

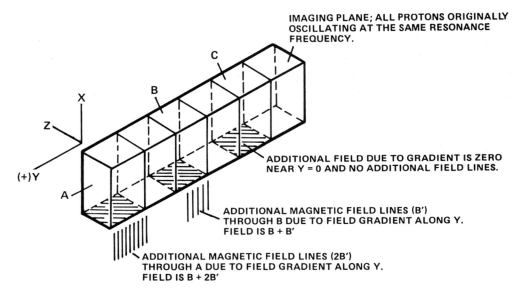

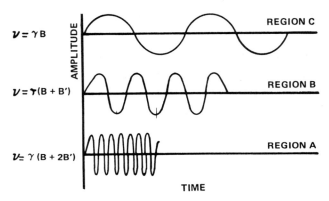

FIG. 2-4. For protons already at resonance in a narrow plane, an additional linear field gradient along y can frequency encode position in the plane along the y axis.

netic dipole system of Fig. 2-4, if we impose a linear gradient such that the magnetic field increases along the (+) y direction, the *oscillation frequencies* of the *already excited* proton dipoles will also increase linearly along the +y direction. This is diagrammed in Fig. 2-4. Near Y = 0, a narrow plane C is near the original oscillation frequency because the magnetic field is near the original field. The field gradient introduces additional magnetic flux through plane B and the oscillation frequencies of those protons are correspondingly greater. The protons in plane A oscillate at the highest frequencies because the magnetic field gradient along y produces the highest magnetic field at A.

We have outlined a magnetic resonance method for specifying the location of proton magnetic dipoles in tissue along the z axis and along the y axis. That is, we can obtain a projection of the proton density in the zy plane (cross-hatched area in Fig. 2-4). If the x location could be specified using another magnetic resonance parameter, a two-dimensional image could be constructed. This additional parameter, phase, is considered in the next sections.

2.4 Oscillating Magnetic Fields and Electrical Currents: The Concept of Phase

The concept of the phase of the oscillation of magnetic dipoles is central to the understanding of how proton magnetic resonance images (MRIs) are constructed. A simple experimentally verifiable model of phase is illustrated in Fig. 2-5. The time dependencies of the voltages in the two circuits are 180° *out of phase* because the bar magnet oscillations are out of phase by that amount. As shown before, one complete pattern of the time dependence of the voltage change, after which the pattern repeats itself, is called one cycle, which is 360°, as shown in Diagram 2-2.

Diagram 2-3 depicts the time dependencies of the voltage changes for two identical magnetic oscillators out of phase (phase shifted) by various angles and the resultant net voltage changes with time. Note that the voltage for in-phase oscillators is twice as large as that for the individual oscillators. For example, this would be the case in the circuit of Fig. 2-5 if both bar magnets were forced to undergo oscillation from the same starting point, i.e., the -1 position. For this in-phase oscillation, the current is forced to flow in the same direction in each loop at any given time.

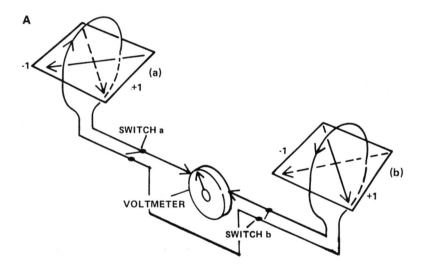

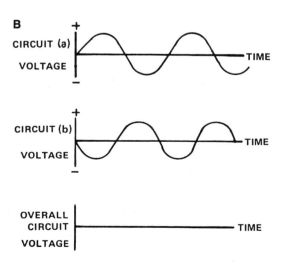

FIG. 2-5. **A:** Two isolated bar magnets oscillating through two connected wire loops. The bar magnets are identical and oscillate at the same frequency. Magnet (a) is oriented toward -1 and magnet (b) is oriented toward $+1$ and held. Both magnets are released simultaneously and the direction of the flow of current at the instant the bar magnets swing through 0 is shown. Since the flow, if it could occur, is opposed at the meter, there is no net flow of electricity in the circuit and no voltage change. **B:** The dependency of voltage change that would occur in isolated circuits (sampled by alternately opening and closing the appropriate switches). If we open both switches so that the circuits are not isolated, there will be *no overall* voltage change with time because the magnet oscillations are *out of phase* and so is the alternating current. The voltages in fact are 180° *out of phase*.

DIAGRAM 2-2. One cycle comprises 360°.

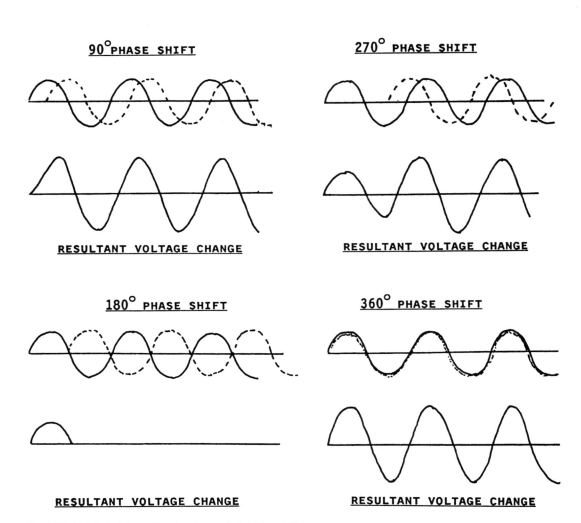

DIAGRAM 2-3. Two signals phase shifted by different angles.

2.5 Phase Encoding of Position with a Third Orthogonal Field Gradient Along the X Coordinate

The receiver coils and detection system used in proton MRI can measure not only the frequency but also the *phase* of the signal generated by the oscillating magnetic dipole. Phase-sensitive detectors are used and with the aid of computers, it is straightforward to separate a complex mixture of phase-shifted signals of different frequencies into individual signals characterized by a unique frequency and phase. It is thus possible to use the signal phase to encode its position by the use of a linear magnetic field gradient. We can outline how this might be accomplished with the aid of Fig. 2-6. In Panel I of the figure we have sketched proton magnetic dipoles at resonance at 1.00000 T in a plane preselected along the z axis by methods outlined in the previous section. They are at four different locations, a,b,c,d, along the x axis that have the same resonance frequency of 42.6 MHz or 42,600,000 cycles/sec. The protons are oscillating in phase, each starting at +1, moving to −1, and back to +1, completing each such cycle in 1/42,600,000 sec, and collectively introducing four times the voltage change of a single proton in the receiver coil.

Now suppose that we turn on, as in Panel II, a linear field gradient of 2 G or 0.0002 T/cm along the x axis for the short time of 0.1 msec (0.0001 sec). As shown in Panel II, the gradient is imposed such that proton (a) continues to be in a field of 1.00000 T but that protons (b), (c), and (d) experience a linearly varying field; e.g., the field at (d) is 1.00000 T + 0.0002 T/cm × 2 cm = 1.0004 T. The resonance frequency of proton (a) continues to be 42.6 MHz ($v = \gamma B = 42.6 \times 1.0000$), but the resonance frequency of (d) now is $v = \gamma B = 42.6 \times 1.0004 = 42.617$ MHz. The

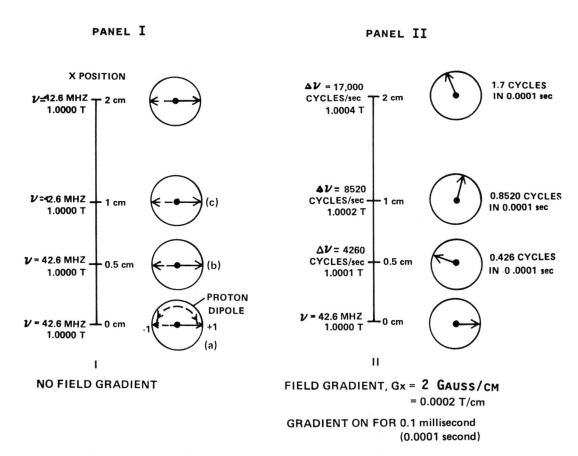

FIG. 2-6. Time dependence of phase changes of proton dipoles in field gradients turned on for different times: Panel I, gradient off; panel II, gradient turned on for 0.1 msec; panel III, gradient on for 0.5 msec; and panel IV, gradient on for 1.0 msec.

FIG. 2-6. *Continued next page.*

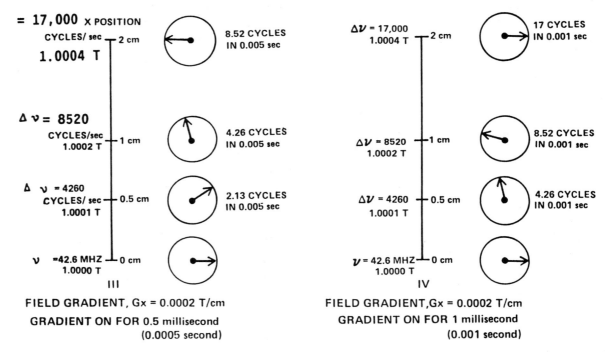

FIG. 2-6. *Continued.*

difference in the resonance frequencies of (a) and (d) Δυ is 0.0170 MHz or 17,000 Hz (cycles/sec). The differences in the resonance frequencies between proton (a) and protons (b), (c), (d) are given in Fig. 2-6 for each of the times that the field gradient is left on.

What is the consequence of turning the field gradient on for a time as short as even 0.1 msec (0.0001 sec)? As shown in the figure, proton dipoles (b), (c), and (d) will change phase with respect to proton (a) because they are oscillating faster; e.g., proton (b) is resonating 4260 cycles/sec faster than proton (a) (Panel II) and in 0.0001 second will have gained 0.426 cycles of oscillation, while protons (c) and (d) will have gained 0.852 and 1.7 cycles respectively. Since the detectors we use in proton MRI are tuned to the resonance frequency (42.6 MHz for a 1.00000-T field) and locked to the phase of the oscillation, the detector will sense the average phase or phase shift of the protons after the field gradient is turned off. (These are shown in Diagram 2-6 using projection methods similar to those of Fig. 2-2.) Note that the magnetic dipoles add as vectors, as shown in Diagram 2-4, and the detector cannot distinguish dipoles that have completed 0, 1, or n × 1 cycles of oscillation so that 1.7 cycles of phase shift is equivalent to a 0.7-cycle phase shift and a 17-cycle phase shift is equivalent to a 0 cycle phase shift. The cycles are defined in Diagrams 2-5 and 2-6.

If a sufficient number of average phases is obtained by turning the gradient along x on a sufficient number of different times, then a computer can be used to assign a relative phase to each position along the x axis. Although the computer manipulations are complex, the physical bases for the results are reasonable: as the x coordinate increases, the phase change

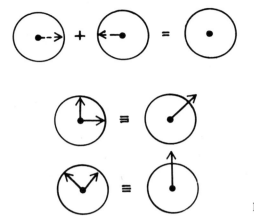

DIAGRAM 2-4. Vector addition.

0.25, 1.25...CYCLES
0.5, 1.5,...CYCLES
0, 1, 2...CYCLES

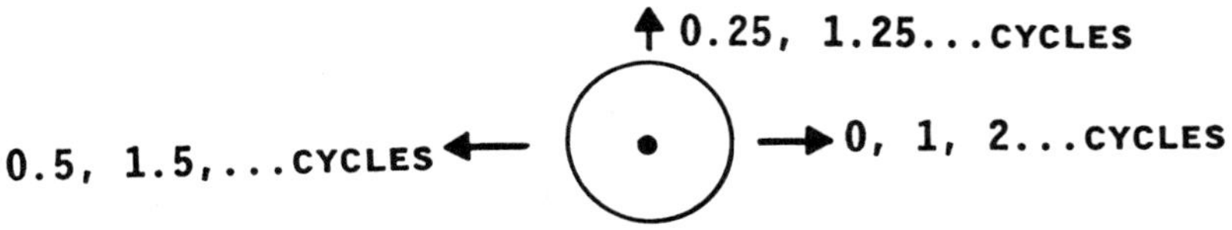

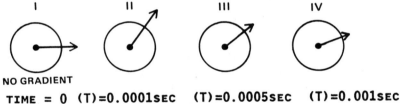

DIAGRAM 2-5. Definition of cycles in the model described.

I
II
III
IV
NO GRADIENT
TIME = 0
(T)=0.0001SEC
(T)=0.0005SEC
(T)=0.001SEC

DIAGRAM 2-6. Average phases of the proton dipoles subjected to the field gradients described in panels I, II, III, and IV of Fig. 2-6.

increases because of the increase in the magnetic field due to the gradient, and the large number of times the gradients must be turned on, to disentangle the relative phase information, resides in the lack of information in many of the individual phase shifts.

2.6 The Central Theme of Proton Magnetic Resonance Imaging is That the Application of Three Orthogonal Field Gradients to Proton Magnetic Dipoles in a Static (Orienting) Magnetic Field Can be Used to Define the Location (X, Y, Z Coordinates) of Proton Density: The Precise Order in Which the Gradients are Applied is Critical to Putting It All Together

A proton MRI is a three-dimensional map of the proton concentration (density) in body water and fat molecules in the spatial coordinates x,y,z (length, width, height). The proton concentration is assessed indirectly through measurements of the magnetization acquired by proton nuclear magnetic dipoles in a static (orienting) field. The measurements are made by first applying a second magnetic field which, at resonance, tips the net proton magnetization out of alignment with the static field. Then the oscillatory realignment of the magnetization is detected with a sensitive receiver coil. The net magnetization detected is proportional to the proton concentration in the volume of observation. The spatial coordinates of the volume observed can be defined by imposing linear field gradients along the x,y, and z axes so that the frequency and phase of the proton resonances become a linear function of the x,y, and z positions. In the model we have chosen for proton MRI the following specific sequence of events occurs (Fig. 2-7):

—the patient is placed in a magnet that quickly orients the proton magnetic dipoles (A)

—a field gradient is imposed on the z axis such that a narrow (3 mm–1 cm) selected plane of protons resonate within a narrow band of selected frequencies (B)

—with the z field gradient still on, a transmitter coil operating at the selected frequency excites the protons in the selected plane to resonance. The z gradient and the transmitter are turned off, and the protons in the plane continue to oscillate (C)

—a field gradient along the x axis is turned on for a short time and then it is turned off. During the time it is turned on, the dipoles along the x coordinate acquire different phases of oscillation, those at the largest field (with the largest x coordinate) acquire the largest phase shift (D)

—a field gradient is now turned on along the y axis to frequency encode position of the dipoles (which are already at resonance) and simultaneously a receiver coil is turned on to record the signals (E). Normally, 128, 265, or 512 data points along the frequency encoding axis are recorded. The larger is the number of data points, the higher the resolution.

—because we detect only the average phase of the protons in the plane

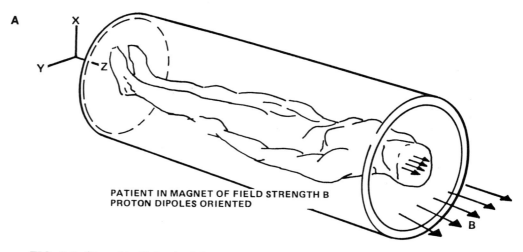

FIG. 2-7. Steps (A–E) in obtaining a proton MRI.

Mapping Proton Density in The xy Plane

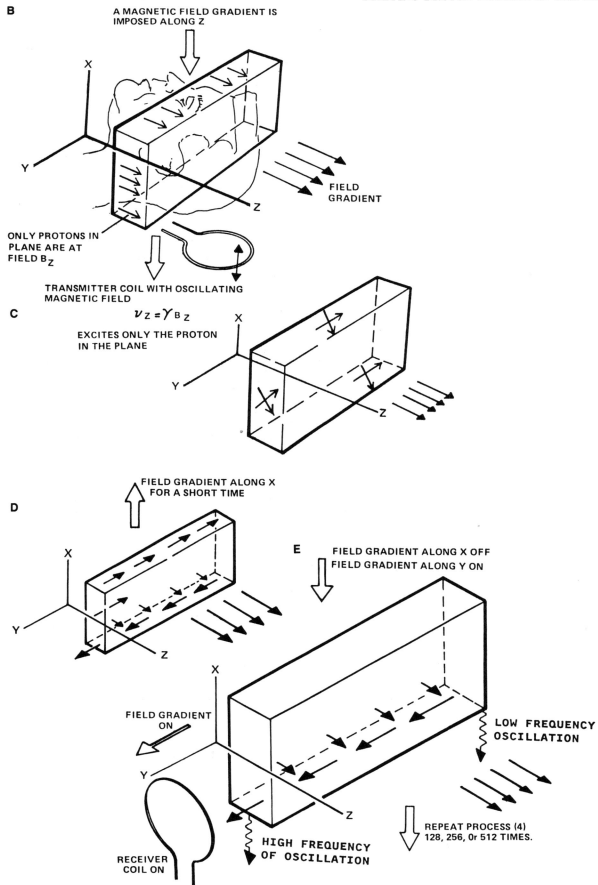

excited, we must repeat the process (D) many times to fix accurately the positions of the proton dipoles along the x axis. Mathematically, to achieve a resolution along x that is equal to that along y, we must apply different values of the phase-encoding gradient for a total number of different times that is equal to the number of frequency encoding data points, e.g., 128, 256, or 512. Alternatively, and this is what is usually done, the phase-encoding gradient *amplitude* (value of G/cm) can be changed, keeping the time the gradient is applied constant; changing the gradient amplitude in a stepwise fashion has an effect on the phase that is equivalent to keeping the amplitude constant, but changing the length of time the gradient is on.

2.7 Shorthand Notation for the Processes in Proton Magnetic Resonance Imaging: A Simplified Timing Diagram

A shorthand notation for the processes discussed in Section 2.6 is shown in Diagram 2-7. Note that we have illustrated the processes involved in proton imaging by selecting an imaging plane (slice) along the z axis which is the long axis of the body. The slice selected is in the xy plane, the so-called axial plane. The gradient functions are easily switched and the slice selection gradient could be applied along the y axis, in which case the imaging plane would be the zx or sagittal plane. Similarly, if G_x were used for slice selection, the plane imaged would be the zy or coronal plane.

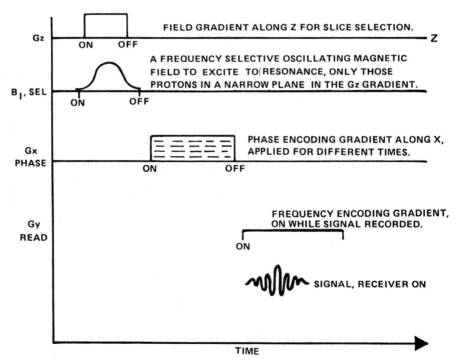

DIAGRAM 2-7. A simplified timing diagram.

QUESTIONS FOR CHAPTER 2

Pick out the one false statement for each of the following:

1. The proton magnetic resonance signal:
   - can be expressed in units of cycles/sec or Hz, or in larger units, MHz
   - can be represented by a sine or cosine wave
   - results from the voltage induced in a radiofrequency (RF) coil by the oscillation of proton nuclear dipoles at resonance
   - has a phase that cannot be shifted or altered

2. Essential elements in the overall process of exciting to resonance only the protons in the imaging slice desired include:
   - applying a linear gradient along the static magnetic field
   - applying a selective RF pulse whose narrow range of frequencies excites to resonance only those protons in a known location in the magnetic field gradient
   - moving the patient in the bore of the magnet so that the RF coil can excite a specific slice of protons

3. The phase of a proton magnetic resonance signal:
   - can be changed by changing for a short time the strength of the magnetic field experienced by protons already at resonance in the selected slice
   - can specify the spatial location of the protons in the excited slice if the phase is altered by the imposition of a linear field gradient for a known short time after excitation of the protons to resonance
   - is the same as that for the signal of a proton that has experienced a 360° phase shift owing to the imposition of a field gradient
   - is the same as that for the signal of a proton that has experienced a 180° phase shift owing to the imposition of a field gradient

4. The frequency of a proton magnetic resonance signal:
   - can be changed by the strength of the magnetic field experienced by protons already at resonance in the selected slice
   - can specify the spatial location of the protons in the excited slice if a known linear static magnetic field gradient is imposed while the magnetic resonance signals of the excited slice are being acquired
   - can be changed by the RF oscillator
   - depends on the strength of the static magnet field including that contributed by linear gradients of that field

5. The phase and frequency of a proton magnetic resonance signal:
   - cannot be changed after the protons in the imaging slice selected have been excited to resonance
   - are the two parameters that can be used to define the spatial location of protons in the imaging slice excited to resonance
   - contain a record of the history of the magnetic fields, magnetic field gradients, and RF excitation to which a tissue has been subjected
   - can both be determined in a proton MRI study

3

Components of Proton Magnetic Resonance Imaging Systems

The major components of proton imaging systems include: a large bore magnet capable of accepting a human torso and having a homogeneous magnetic field that orients the proton dipoles in human tissue; a set of large coils for generating known linear gradients of the magnetic field in the x,y, and z directions; a transceiver system for transmitting the oscillating magnetic fields to excite protons to resonance and for receiving the proton magnetic resonance signals; and a computer system for processing the magnetic resonance signals into an image. In this chapter we will explore key features of these system components, which are sketched in Fig. 3-1.

3.1 The Shape of the Fields of Some Permanent Magnets

The reality of the force fields of magnets has been illustrated in the first two chapters using examples common to our experience. The shape of the fields of *permanent* magnets and their dependence on magnet geometry is illustrated in Fig. 3-2. The fields can be readily visualized by scattering iron filings (or ferrite particles) on a stiff piece of paper and placing the magnet under the paper. The filings will align themselves parallel to the magnetic field lines. The situation depicted in Fig. 3-2C is especially interesting—the magnetic field lines between the two bar magnets near the center are parallel. This is called a homogeneous magnetic field, a condition we strive for in the magnets used in proton magnetic resonance imaging (MRI). By a very homogeneous magnetic field we mean, e.g., that if the

32 MAGNETIC RESONANCE WORKBOOK

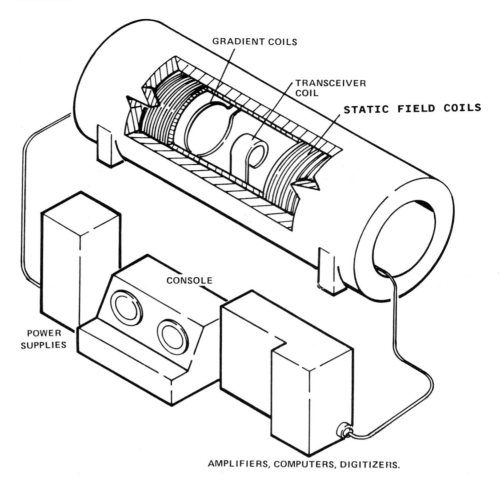

FIG. 3-1. Components of a proton MRI system.

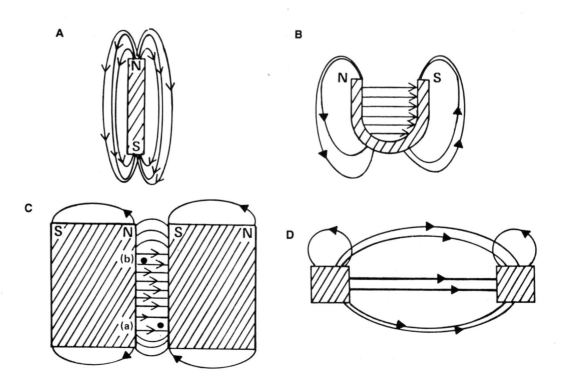

field at point A (Fig. 3-2C) is 1.000000 T, then the field at point B should also be 1.000000 T. If such is the case, then the proton resonance frequencies at the two points will be exactly 42.5759 MHz ($v = \gamma B$, where γ for the proton is actually 42.5759 MHz/T). Since, in many magnetic resonance studies, the resolution of our measurements must be better than one cycle (0.000001 MHz), the magnetic field over the volume of our measurement must be correspondingly homogeneous.

Another important aspect of magnetic fields is illustrated in Fig. 3-2D: as the poles of the magnets move farther and farther away, the strength of the field *between the poles* decreases and, not coincidentally, the area of homogeneity of the field between the poles decreases.

3.2 Permanent Magnets for Low-Field Proton Magnetic Resonance Imaging

As discussed in Section 1.2, some materials can become permanently magnetized when subjected to a strong magnetic field. The origin of this permanent magnetization is the parallel alignment by the magnetic field of domains in the structure, which are tiny circuits of moving electrons (permanent electrical currents). These domains remain aligned after the external magnetic field is removed. Materials that exhibit this behavior are ferromagnetic and include substances such as iron, nickel, cobalt, alloys of these metals, and certain oxides, such as ferrite. The most intense magnetic fields within ferromagnetic materials with complete alignment of the domains is approximately 1 T. When fabricated into permanent magnets like that sketched in Fig. 3-3, the magnetic field in the space occupied by the patient is reduced to ~0.05 T because the magnet poles must be separated by a large distance.

The low fields intrinsic to permanent magnets have limited their use in proton MRI. In the low fields, tissue becomes very slightly magnetized, the proton resonance signals are faint, and long times are required to obtain acceptable data, even in relatively thick (1 cm) imaging planes. Low-field magnets are now being considered more seriously for proton imaging in trauma units because the low magnetic fields and forces involved allow the use of steel oxygen bottles and life-support systems that would become deadly projectiles in the fringe fields of 0.35 to 1.5 T imaging systems. Marked improvements in the technology for fabricating highly sensitive receiver coils have led to the reconsideration of these low-field magnets and their use in special applications.

FIG. 3-2. Magnetic field lines (fluxes) of permanent magnets. **A:** A bar magnet. **B:** A horseshoe magnet. **C:** Two close bar magnets with opposite poles facing. **D:** Two distant bar magnets with opposite poles facing.

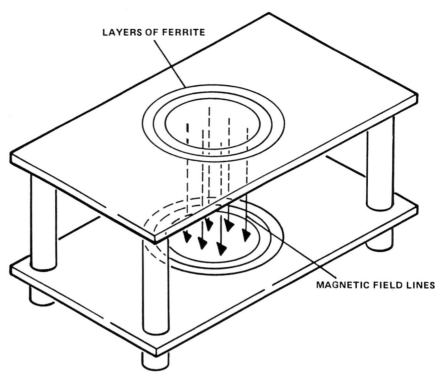

FIG. 3-3. Permanent magnet composed of layers of magnetized ferrite. The magnetic field runs parallel to the columns between which the patient's bed slides.

3.3 Magnetic Fields of Wires Carrying Electrical Current

The magnetic fields attainable with a ferromagnetic material are limited by the number of natural current-carrying domains in the material and how well they can be aligned. In contrast, with a large electromotive force (voltage), we can force large amounts of electrical current to flow through coils of conducting wires. The magnetic fields in the center of such coils are correspondingly large. In fact, working magnetic fields as large as 12 T have been used routinely in nuclear magnetic resonance (NMR) studies by passing electrical current through coils of special materials at low temperatures. The shapes of the magnetic fields of current-conducting coils are central to understanding the magnets used in most proton MRI systems. The evolution of a magnetic field from the circular one of a linear wire to the linear one of tightly wound loops is sketched in Fig. 3-4. The key feature of the evolution is that when a wire is wound into a series of loops, the magnetic fields of the segments of the loops can reinforce (add to each other, point in the same direction) or cancel each other. In a long, tightly wound solenoid (Fig. 3-4D), this results in parallel, evenly spaced lines in the interior of the solenoid, i.e., a homogeneous magnetic field.

There is a price to pay for the homogeneous magnetic field in the interior of a long, tightly wound solenoid: large magnetic fields, called fringe fields, exist far from the center of the coil. For a 0.5 T coil which is 2.3 m long and 1 m in diameter, the fringe fields are large, as illustrated in Diagram

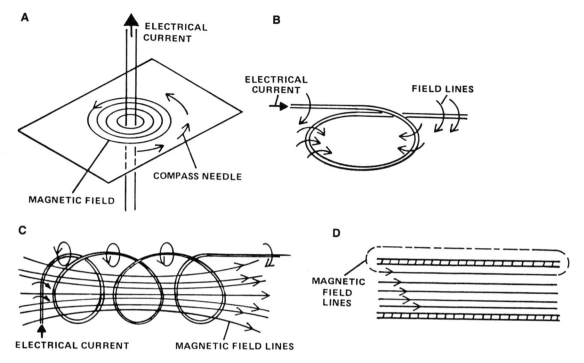

FIG. 3-4. Magnetic field lines (fluxes) of wire carrying electrical current. **A:** Long linear wire. **B:** Loop of wire. **C:** Loosely wound solenoid. **D:** Very long solenoid, tightly wound. Electrical current goes out of the paper at the top and into the paper at the bottom.

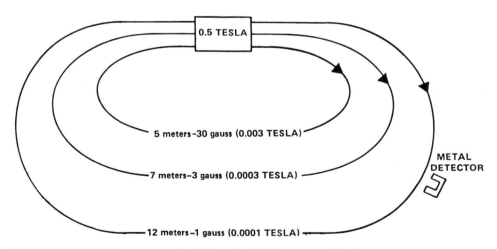

DIAGRAM 3-1. Fringe magnetic fields of a 0.5-T superconducting magnet.

3-1. The large fringe fields at a distance increase siting costs and safety precautions because fringe fields of:

  –30 G affect the operation of computers
  –3 G affect the operation of television monitors
  –5–10 G affect the operation of some pacemakers
  –large steel objects such as gas cylinders will be accelerated to the center
of the field by a fringe field of ~30 Gauss.

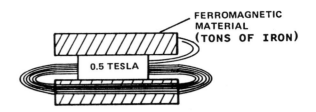

DIAGRAM 3-2. Concentration of fringe magnetic fields with a ferromagnetic shield.

Magnetic field lines concentrate in ferromagnetic materials compared to air so that fringe fields can be reduced by placing ferromagnetic shields around the magnet, as shown in Diagram 3-2. Shielded solenoids are in common use, but the shields may adversely affect magnetic field homogeneity in some proton magnetic resonance studies.

3.4 Resistive Electromagnets with an Iron Core

Electromagnets with iron cores, such as those sketched in Fig. 3-5, provide convenient short paths through the iron cores for the magnetic fields generated by the electric current flowing in the coils. This markedly reduces the fringe fields and results in homogeneous magnetic fields over the large volumes examined in proton MRI. The magnetic fields generated not only by the current flowing in the coils, but also by the alignment of

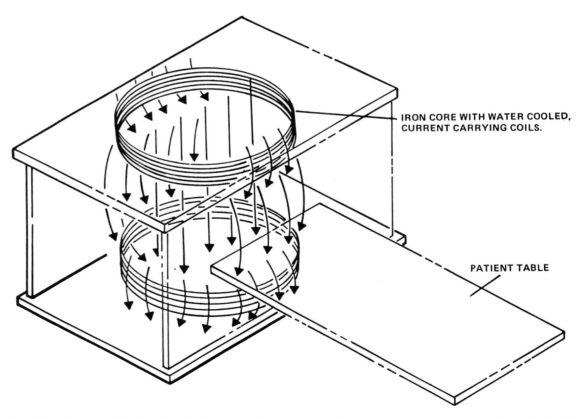

FIG. 3-5. Sketch of part of an electromagnet. The essential iron yoke of such a magnet has been deleted for simplicity.

the domains in the ferromagnetic material, can be quite large. When the N and S poles of such a magnet are separated by only a few mm the field can be as large as 2.0 T. When the N and S poles are separated by 50 cm or more to allow patient access, the maximum practical homogeneous field attainable is ~0.5 T. Even that field requires extremely high electrical currents (hundreds of amps) through the coils and the heat generated by the resistance of the coils (power dissipation, tens of Kilowatts) requires a closed circuit water cooling of the coils with an associated water chiller system. The magnets are very heavy, 7 to 13 tons depending on the field strength.

3.5 Superconducting Magnets

Superconductors are materials that have no electrical resistivity and can conduct large amounts of electrical current without power loss in resistance heating. This property is characteristic of a limited class of metals and alloys (niobium/titanium, NbTi; niobium/tin, Nb_3Sn; and vanadium/gallium, V_3Ga) at very low temperatures, near the boiling point of liquid helium (~4° K or ~ −269° C). Wires made of a superconductor like NbTi can be wound into solenoids that can conduct extremely high densities of electricity at liquid helium temperatures and generate intense homogeneous magnetic fields (0.5–2.0 T) over large volumes (1 m diameter). Fig. 3-6 shows a superconducting magnet that is essentially a fiber-reinforced

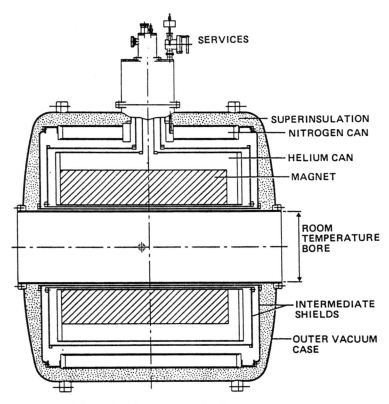

FIG. 3-6. Schematic of a superconducting magnet.

DIAGRAM 3-3. Superconducting wires are imbedded in a low electrical resistance copper matrix.

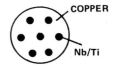

epoxy tube around which the superconducting wire is coiled and cemented with epoxy. The bulk of the magnet assembly consists of a cryostat that provides a constant low temperature environment to maintain the superconductor at liquid helium temperatures in an economical manner. Consequently, the cryostat must be well insulated and constructed of material with a low thermal conductivity. A reservoir with a bath of liquid nitrogen (boiling point 77° K) and liquid helium, rather than liquid helium alone, is used to maintain the temperature because helium is expensive and has a low heat capacity. Liquid nitrogen is a factor of 10 less in cost and absorbs 60 times as much heat as liquid helium when it evaporates. A well designed cryostat for a 1-m bore 1.5 T magnet will result in boil off rates of ~0.35 L/hr for helium and 0.65 L/hr for nitrogen.

A superconducting magnet can rapidly deenergize or "quench" when a region of the solenoid windings become resistive by local heating, which drives the local temperature above the superconducting temperature. Local heating can be caused by friction from mechanical vibrations or through a fall in the level of liquid helium coolant. The resistance heating can propagate rapidly throughout the bulk of the windings, resulting in a rapid boil-off of the coolants accompanied by a loud noise. For this and other technical reasons, the NbTi conductors are imbedded in a copper matrix which has a high thermal conductivity and a very low electrical resistivity, as shown in Diagram 3-3. The copper provides a low resistance (low heating) path for the current if the NbTi alloy is temporarily driven above the superconducting temperature.

The favorable aspects of superconducting magnets that have led to their widespread acceptance for proton imaging systems include:

–fields as large as 4 T can be created over volumes having a diameter as large as 1 m
–very homogeneous fields can be created
–once the magnet has been energized, the field is a persistent one if the right kind of electrical switch is employed. After the energization the power supply can be removed
–operating costs are reasonable.

The disadvantages of superconducting magnets include:

–high capital cost of the magnet
–the large fringe fields that increase siting costs and the complexity of safety procedures
–liquid nitrogen and helium coolants must be replenished on a periodic basis.

3.6 Coils for Creating Linear Gradients in the Strength of the Static Field

The homogeneous static magnetic field depicted in Fig. 3-7A might be generated by a long coil homogeneously and tightly wound as in Fig. 3-4. If inside the long homogeneous coil, a much looser coil is placed with a gradient in the number of turns and with current running in different directions on the opposite ends of the coil (Fig. 3-7B), then a linear gradient in the static magnetic field can be created, as shown in Fig. 3-7C. The strength of the field gradient (G/cm) is a function of the current and number of windings in the gradient coil. The maximum easily attainable gradients are approximately 2 G (0.0002 T)/cm for 1-m bore magnet. The strength of the field gradients affects the slice thickness, field of view, and resolution.

The coils shown in Fig. 3-7B are for creating a gradient along the main axis of the magnet coil, conventionally defined as the z direction. Coils for creating gradients along the x and y directions are more complex and have a Golay, or saddle geometry. To save space, the gradient coils are put as a single assembly inside the magnet bore, where they are energized individually for short periods of time (a few msec) during the imaging procedure. Thus, an important additional design consideration for gradient coils is the rise time of the power amplifier that "drives" them.

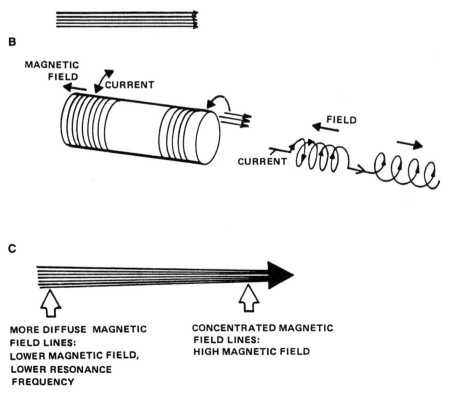

FIG. 3-7. Magnetic field gradients. A: Static homogeneous magnetic field. B: Gradient coil. C: Magnetic field with linear gradient.

3.7 Magnet Shimming

It is very difficult to wind a "perfect" coil for creating a static field that is as homogeneous as required for proton MRI. Even if the perfect coil were made, most NMR sites are not magnetically pristine, e.g., devoid of iron objects that can distort the magnetic field. To improve the homogeneity of a magnet in place, a process called shimming is used. As shown in Section 3.3, iron objects tend to concentrate the lines of magnetic flux, i.e., iron has a higher magnetic permeability than air. If a magnet is placed in a site containing structural steel, the field will be distorted by the steel. The field can be passively shimmed by the strategic placement of additional iron to offset the effects. Symmetrical passive shimming, illustrated in Fig. 3-8, is difficult to achieve in practice. Passive shimming in a magnetically contaminated site (or a magnet with poor homogeneity to start with) is accomplished by iteration with the aid of computer modeling and may require placing small pieces of iron on the deenergized magnet itself.

The final adjustments of the magnet homogeneity are accomplished by active shimming with shim coils placed in the bore between the main coils and the gradient coils. These coils, when energized with small amounts of electrical current, add or subtract the proper amounts of field in the proper spaces to render the main field homogeneous as measured by monitoring the range of the proton resonance frequency in space.

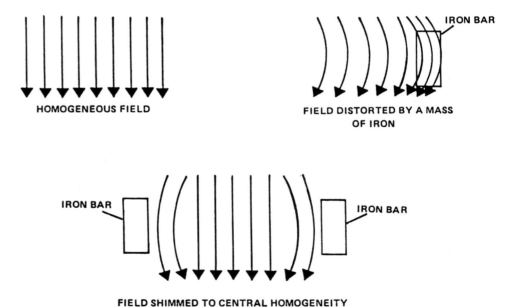

FIG. 3-8. Distortion and passive shimming of a static magnetic field by pieces of iron.

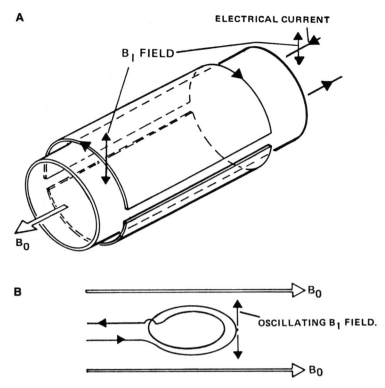

FIG. 3-9. RF coils. **A:** Body coil, saddle-shaped. **B:** Surface coil, for spine imaging. The person would recline on the coil in the magnetic field. The long axis of the body is parallel to B_0 and the coil creates an oscillating B_1 perpendicular to B_0.

3.8 Radiofrequency Coils

The coils used to transmit the oscillating magnetic fields to excite proton dipoles to resonance in a static field or to receive the signal emitted by proton magnetic dipoles at resonance are called radiofrequency (RF) coils because they operate in the MHz range of frequencies characteristic of the oscillation of the *electric dipoles* used in radio. The transmitting and receiving coils must be oriented so that the oscillating magnetic fields they transmit or receive are perpendicular to the static magnetic field along which the proton dipoles are oriented. The coils must also be large enough either to encircle the body part being studied or, if laid on the body surface, to receive NMR signals from the deep-lying structures of the body. RF coils come in all shapes and sizes to accomplish these ends and may be used as both transmitters and receivers.

Fig. 3-9A shows a large body coil that would fit snugly all along the inside bore of a solenoid that already contains tightly fitting gradient and shim coils. The wiring of this body coil is saddle-shaped, allowing the pulse of electrical current to generate a pulse of B_1 oscillating magnetic field which, as shown, is perpendicular to the B_0 field. A smaller radius, shorter coil might be used to obtain proton images of the head alone. An alternative wiring design for these coils resembles a bird cage (bird cage coil), a shape currently popular for body coils on some MRI systems. Recently, attention has been given to special coils for localized imaging of wrist, ankle, elbow, knee, etc. Another special type of coil, a surface coil (Fig. 3-9B), has been in widespread use for imaging the spine and other structures close to the body surface. The reason for the profusion of RF coil types is to improve the sensitivity of an inherently insensitive method.

RF coil design and construction is a highly skilled art and the detailed technical considerations involved in improving the sensitivity of coils is beyond the scope of the discussion here. One aspect of the use of RF coils, however, is straightforward—the closer the coil is to the object being imaged, the more signal is detected per unit volume. Thus it may be necessary to use a large body coil to image the torso, but it is intuitively obvious that, other things being equal, a smaller head coil will provide more signal for head images than will a body coil used for the same purpose. It is less obvious, but equally true, that a surface coil will provide improved spine images compared to a body coil. In this case, for technical reasons, the body coil might serve as a transmitter and the surface coil as a receiver. The price paid for improved images of the spine with a surface coil is that volume of its sensitivity is roughly equal to its dimensions, and acquiring images of the complete spine would require moving the coil several times, or using a matrix of these coils.

The signal intensity discriminated by the RF coil also depends on the electronic noise in the coil. The noise can come from external sources (e.g., radio stations), which can be eliminated by RF shielding, e.g., by enclosing the magnet room with a screen of metallic conductorlike copper. Even with RF shielding, there is noise in the copper RF coil itself because of the thermal motion of electrons in the coil. Not much can be done about this, or probably should be done because a larger source of RF noise in the magnet room is the patient himself, whose tissue contains large quantities of conducting ions. The currents of conducting ions in tissue can create resistance in the coil.

3.9 Computer Requirements

Details of computer requirements for MRI systems will be considered in another workbook. Here we note only that MRI generates large data sets that have stringent computer requirements. For example, one type of imaging procedure acquires serial data from as many as 20 imaging planes containing information in 256×256 phase- and frequency-encoded matrices with a resolution of ~ 1 mm $\times$ 1 mm $\times$ 3 mm. The size of this data set is more than 24,000,000 bytes of information. Sometimes, for technical reasons, eight data sets are collected for each imaging plane in a single diagnostic procedure, which requires ~ 30 minutes alone to collect the complete data set. Added to, or interspersed with, this collection is the time required for tape archiving and filming of the images. It is not surprising then that the computer specifications for a typical proton imaging system include a minicomputer with 2 MB of main memory containing 32 bit words, a floating point array processor for preprocessing data and image reconstruction, and twin disc drives, each with 354 MB capacity.

QUESTIONS FOR CHAPTER 3

Pick out the one false statement for each of the following:

1. A proton magnetic resonance imaging system includes the following components:
   - a wide bore, strong magnet with gradient coils
   - a microcomputer for processing large data sets
   - a transceiver system for exciting protons to resonance and detecting and amplifying the proton magnetic resonance signal
   - a display console

2. Magnets for proton imaging systems:
   - must be constructed with superconducting wires
   - must be reasonably homogeneous
   - must be large enough to contain the body part being imaged
   - affect the quality of the images and the time required to obtain them

3. Magnet shimming:
   - is best done at the factory, especially if the imaging site contains large masses of iron near the 5 G line of the magnet
   - can be accomplished with electrical coils
   - can be accomplished by strategic placement of pieces of iron on or near the magnets
   - improves the homogeneity of the magnet

4. In site planning, considerations of the fringe magnetic fields are important because fringe fields greater than 5 to 30 G can affect:
   - computers
   - cathode ray tubes (monitors)
   - pacemakers
   - human nerves

4

The Proton as a Three-Dimensional Oscillator

4.1 Introduction

In Chapters 1 and 2 the behavior of a proton magnetic dipole oriented in a static magnetic field and perturbed by an oscillating field at right angles to the static field has been described by considering the proton magnetic dipole as a two-dimensional (2D) oscillator like a compass needle. This 2D model, though conceptually simple, cannot be used to describe satisfactorily the time dependence of processes that have a pronounced effect on the appearance and information content of proton magnetic resonance images (MRIs). Accordingly, in this chapter, we extend the description of the oscillations of protons in magnetic fields to three dimensions, beginning with the concept of spin. In Chapters 5 and 6, we use the three-dimensional (3D) model to explore the time dependence of proton magnetization and its influence on the manipulation of intensity and contrast in proton MRI.

4.2 Concept of Spin: Classical

Like many atomic nuclei of biological interest, the proton exhibits a property called spin, associated with which are nuclear angular momentum and a nuclear magnetic moment. A classical picture of spin and magnetic moment and angular momentum associated with the spinning of a charged mass is illustrated in Fig. 4-1. The moving charge of the nucleus of the proton is an electrical current that has an associated magnetic field which is represented by the magnetic moment, "μ". A spinning mass has an

45

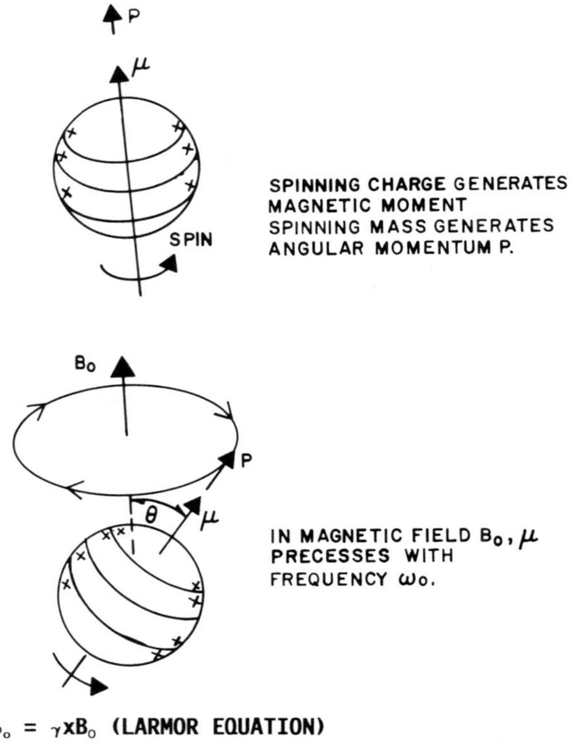

SPINNING CHARGE GENERATES MAGNETIC MOMENT
SPINNING MASS GENERATES ANGULAR MOMENTUM P.

IN MAGNETIC FIELD B_0, μ PRECESSES WITH FREQUENCY ω_0.

FIG. 4-1. Classical models of proton spin, angular momentum, and magnetic moment: The precession of the proton dipole about the static field B_0.

$$\omega_0 = \gamma \mathbf{x} B_0 \quad \textbf{(LARMOR EQUATION)}$$

angular momentum denoted by "P". The magnetic moment of the proton causes it to tend to align with a static magnetic field as we have shown before, but the angular momentum of the proton ensures that the proton magnetic moment will not be motionless in the static field, but will precess about the field direction with a characteristic frequency, the Larmor frequency:

$$\omega_0 = \gamma B_0$$

The motion of a spinning top in the earth's gravitational field provides a simple analogy for appreciating why precession occurs.

If a rapidly spinning top is pushed from its alignment with the earth's gravitational field, it will wobble or precess about the original axis because gravitation exerts a force on the spinning mass. The occurrence of precessional motion in response to the force reflects one of Newton's Laws—when a force is exerted on a spinning object, it tends to move not in the direction of the force, but at right angles to the force. The top does not fall over, it precesses.

In the case of the proton magnetic dipole, the force is exerted by the magnetic field and precession results from the force, the spin, and the lack of perfect alignment of the proton dipole with the static magnetic field in the first place. Unlike a compass needle, the proton dipole does not become perfectly aligned even in the strongest fields imaginable because its magnetic moment is quantized, a subject that will be treated in subsequent texts. The precessional frequency of the proton ω_0 is related to the force (the magnetic field strength B_0) through the constant γ which relates the constant magnetic moment of the proton to its constant angular momentum, $\gamma = \mu/P$. In the case of the top, the precessional frequency can be changed by changing the rate of its spin before the application of perturbing force. Unlike the top, the γ of the proton is constant, but we can change its precessional frequency by changing the strength of the static magnetic field.

4.3 The Magnetization of the Sample in Three Dimensions: Phase Revisited

In this section we begin to develop 3D models for the net magnetization of tissue and the way it is manipulated in the production of proton MRIs. A standard way to represent the alignment and precession of a proton dipole in the static field B_0 in three dimensions is shown in Fig. 4-2A. By convention, the direction of B_0 is along the z axis which is the long axis, or cylindrical axis, of a superconducting solenoid. The proton magnetic moment "μ" has a magnitude and a direction—it is a vector quantity. As shown in Chapters 1 and 2, vectors can be combined and can be separated

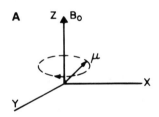

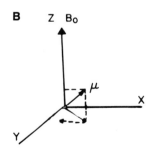

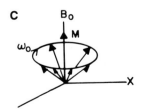

FIG. 4-2. Precession of proton dipoles in a static magnetic field: Static and rotating components. **A:** Single proton dipole, μ precessing about B_0 at the Larmor frequency, $\omega_0 = \gamma B_0$. **B:** Separation of the precessing μ into a static component along B_0 and a component rotating at the frequency ω_0 in the xy plane. **C:** The sample magnetization M is comprised in this case of the sum of the static components of the individual magnetic moments of the sample proton dipoles aligned with the field and precessing about it.

into components for the purpose of simplifying the description of physical processes. The proton magnetic moment can be separated into two components as shown in Fig. 4-2B, a static or motionless component along B_0 or the z axis and a component that rotates in the xy plane at the Larmor frequency. Fig. 4-2B suggests that if we place a radiofrequency (RF) coil in the xy plane and it is tuned to the frequency ω_0, then the component of "μ" rotating in the xy plane should induce an alternating current (voltage) in accordance with Faraday's Laws, as discussed in previous chapters. Note that instead of the oscillation of the moment in the 2D model, in three dimensions the moment rotates a full 360° circle to complete one phase of its motion, inducing current to flow in one direction at 0° and 360° and in the opposite direction at 180°, as illustrated in Diagram 4-1.

The actual method for the generation of the proton resonance signal is more complex because we must consider the motion of all the proton dipoles that align with the field and precess about it at the Larmor frequency, ω_0. As shown in Fig. 4-2C, the sample contains a number of proton dipoles aligned with the field—there are billions of them in tissue samples, but only six are shown for illustrative purposes. The static magnetization M of the sample is a sum of the static components of the individual proton magnetic moments aligned with the field, as shown in Diagram 4-2. As noted in Chapter 1, this net magnetization is weak and almost impossible to detect directly in the presence of the strong field B_0, along which M is aligned. Anticipating the discussion in the next few sections, the detection of the sample magnetization depends on the use of an oscillating RF magnetic field to tilt the magnetization away from alignment along B_0 (z) after which it generates a voltage in a RF receiver coil.

Fig. 4-2C shows *no* net rotating component of magnetization in the xy plane—this is because the individual magnetic moments are precessing with a random phase and the individual components of the proton dipoles rotating in the xy plane cancel the magnetic effects of each other. Recall

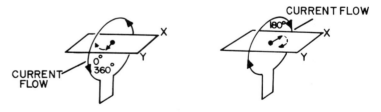

DIAGRAM 4-1. AC induced in a coil by a 360° rotation (precession) of the proton magnetic moment. (In this text we will often denote such an RF coil with the symbol ⌒.)

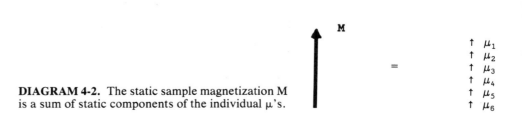

DIAGRAM 4-2. The static sample magnetization M is a sum of static components of the individual μ's.

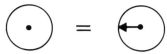

DIAGRAM 4-3. Addition of two vectors 180° out of phase.

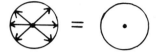

DIAGRAM 4-4. Addition of six vectors out of phase.

that the sum of two vectors of equal magnitude but 180° out of phase is zero, as shown in Diagram 4-3. This is true as well for rotating vectors. As long as the vectors are rotating in the same direction at the same speed, they maintain the 180° phase relationship. For the six proton magnetic moments depicted in Fig. 4-2C, the rotating components of the magnetic moments in the xy plane could be represented, as shown in Diagram 4-4, with *no net* component rotating in the plane because of vector cancellation. Of course these six components merely represent the billions more rotating in the xy plane.

Why is the precession of the proton dipoles characterized by a random phase? Recall from Chapter 1 that the process by which the tissue protons become magnetized is an exponential process lasting a few seconds. The protons that align with the field early in the process will have precessed about the field direction many times compared to protons aligning later in the process, and it would be highly unlikely that the two sets of protons would have the same phase of precession or rotation (i.e., begin each cycle at the same point). Another consideration, perhaps the more important one, is that the proton spins have a random orientation before the application of B_0, and would be expected to become aligned with B_0 at random phases. Also we shall see later that the tissue lattice acts to dephase proton spins once they have been brought into phase with the creation of a signal by the methods discussed in the next sections.

QUESTIONS FOR SECTION 4.3

Complete the statements by circling a choice between the italicized options.

1. The precession of a proton magnetic moment in a static field B_0 can be separated into two components: a motionless or static component aligned along the *x/y/z* axis which coincides with the direction of the B_0/B_1 field; and a component that is *parallel/perpendicular* to the B_0/B_1 field and is rotating at the Larmor frequency.

2. The equilibrium or static magnetization of a sample placed in a static field B_0 is comprised of the *static/rotating* components of the individual magnetic moments.

Continued on page 50.

QUESTIONS FOR SECTION 4.3 continued.

3. The oscillation of the proton magnetic dipole in three dimensions constitutes a full *180°/360°* circle in one phase during which it can induce a *direct/alternating* current in a receiver coil.

4. The tissue proton dipoles oriented by a static B_0 field exhibit no magnetization in the xy plane because the phase of the oriented proton dipoles is *coherent/random*.

4.4 The B_1 Field Creates the Proton Signal: Properties of the Oscillating B_1 Field

As we have noted before, an oscillating B_1 field can be created by passing an alternating current (AC) through a RF coil. As shown in Fig. 4-3A, this field linearly oscillates at right angles to the path of the AC. As the electrical current alternates, the magnetic field oscillates along the y axis in the manner depicted in Diagram 4-5.

Anticipating the next section, what we require to create proton magnetization in the xy plane and hence the proton signal, is a B_1 field that *rotates* at the Larmor frequency. As shown in Fig. 4-3B, one can create a linearly oscillating B_1 field by using two equal-strength B_1 fields rotating at the same frequency but in opposite directions. By the principle of reciprocity discussed in previous chapters, a linearly oscillating field thus can be treated as if it were composed of two B_1 fields rotating in the opposite direction. For reasons that will become obvious in the next section, it is only the B_1 field that rotates in the *same direction* as the precessing proton dipoles that affects the proton magnetization—the B_1 field that is rotating in the opposite direction has no effect and can be neglected.

The B_1 field is characterized by a field strength and a length of time the field is turned on. B_1 fields for proton imaging can be as large as 50 G (0.005 T) and are turned on for as short as 1 μsec (10^{-6} sec) or as long as

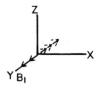

DIAGRAM 4-5. Linearly oscillating B_1 field.

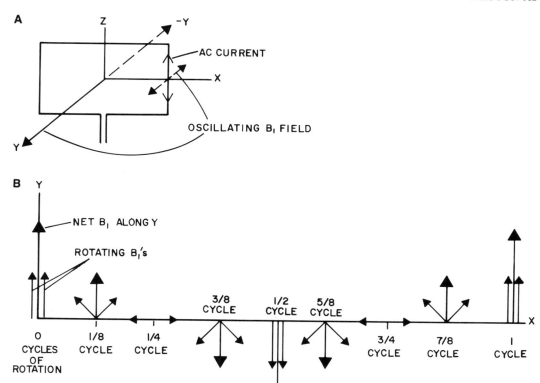

FIG. 4-3. The oscillating B_1 field. **A:** An alternating current passed through a coil generates an oscillating B_1 magnetic field—the current flows in the zx plane and the perpendicular B_1 field is generated along the y axis. **B:** A linear oscillating B_1 field is caused by two B_1 fields rotating in opposite directions.

1 msec (10^{-3} sec). To put these numbers in context, recall that the B_0 field strengths of most imaging systems are 0.5 to 1.5 T and that the length of time required to magnetize biological samples fully is 1 to 4 sec.

QUESTIONS FOR SECTION 4.4

Complete the statements by circling a choice between the italicized options.

1. The passage of an alternating current through a RF coil generates a *static/ oscillating* magnetic field.

2. A linearly oscillating B_1 magnetic field can be created from two *rotating/ stationary* B_1 fields of equal strength.

4.5 Creation of the Proton Signal with an Oscillating Radiofrequency Field: Tilting M Away from B_0 and Creating Phase Coherence in the XY Plane

Consider the component of the B_1 field that is rotating in the same direction as the proton spins are precessing and the B_1 field, of course, is at a right angle to B_0.

If the component is rotating at the Larmor frequency of the proton magnetic dipoles, they experience an additional torque or twisting force from the B_1 magnetic field. The initial conditions immediately after the rotating B_1 field has been turned on is sketched in Fig. 4-4A. Because the B_1 field is rotating at the same frequency as the proton dipoles ω_0, each of the proton dipoles would maintain the same orientation (phase) with respect to B_1 (in the absence of its torque) no matter how many rotations were made about the B_0 axis by the B_1 field and the proton dipoles. An example for one proton dipole is sketched in Diagram 4-6.

At whatever stage of the rotation we inspect the relative orientation of B_1 and μ, it will be the same as viewed down the B_1 axis, i.e., as in Diagram 4-7, where B_0 points up and μ is angled to the right. Thus, as long as B_1 rotates at the same frequency (the Larmor frequency ω_0) as the proton dipoles, then B_1 appears as an additional static field about which the proton dipoles should precess. This is the origin of a torque which, over time, twists the proton dipoles toward the xy plane (Diagram 4-8).

The actual motion of the sample magnetization comprising billions of μ's under the combined influence of the static B_0 and rotating B_1 fields is quite complex. Fig. 4-4B illustrates the spiral course that the tissue magnetization exhibits as it is twisted into the xy plane from its alignment along B_0 during the time that the rotating B_1 field is turned on. After the B_1 field is turned off, the magnetization M will continue to precess about B_0 (this is called free precession) and can generate an alternating current (voltage) in a sensitive receiver coil in the xy plane. This is the proton

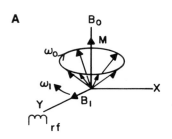

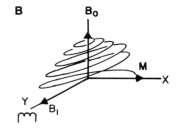

FIG. 4-4. The effect of the B_1 field on the precession of proton dipoles. **A:** Proton dipoles precessing in random phase at ω_0 about B_0 immediately after turning on a B_1 field also rotating at ω_0 ($\omega_1 = \omega_0$). **B:** Spiral course of the evolution of M from *alignment* along B_0 into *rotation* about B_0 under the influence of B_1.

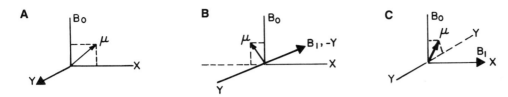

DIAGRAM 4-6. Constant phase between B_1 and μ rotating at ω_0. **A:** Initial state of rotation. **B:** After a half cycle of rotation. **C:** After three-quarter cycle of rotation.

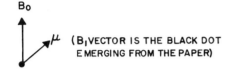

DIAGRAM 4-7. The constant relative orientation of B_1 and μ rotating ω_0, as viewed down the axis of B_1.

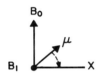

DIAGRAM 4-8. Additional torque or precession of μ about B_1.

magnetic resonance signal. Note that achieving the resonance condition depends on matching exactly the frequencies of the B_1 field and the precessional frequency of the proton dipoles. Without the match, the B_1 field does not maintain phase coherence with the proton dipoles and consequently no persistent torque is exerted on them, no net rotating magnetization is created in the xy plane, and no proton resonance signal is generated. This is also the reason that the effect of the other component of the B_1 field that is rotating in the direction opposite to the direction of precession can be neglected—it cannot maintain a constant phase relationship with the proton dipoles. As discussed in Section 4.6, the rotation of M about B_1 can be simplified considerably by viewing it through the eyes of an observer who is himself rotating at the Larmor frequency.

QUESTIONS FOR SECTION 4.5

Complete the statements by circling a choice between the italicized options.

1. The component of B_1 that rotates in the *same/opposite* direction as (to) the precession of the proton dipoles is used to create phase coherence in the xy plane.

2. After the B_1 field has tipped the magnetization into the xy plane and has been turned off, the magnetization is *stationary/continues to precess about the B_0 field*.

Continued on page 54.

QUESTIONS FOR SECTION 4.5 *continued.*

3. Free precession is described as *rotation of M about B_0 after B_1 has been turned*   *off/the alignment of the proton dipoles with B_0.*

4.6 Rotation of Magnetization by the B_1 Field: Pulse Angles

We can simplify the description of the motion of M under the influence of B_1 by hopping aboard the B_1 vector and viewing the world as from a merry-go-round rotating at the Larmor frequency. In Fig. 4-5A we have sketched what an observer (a detector coil) would see looking down the y axis of a magnetized sample immediately after the RF B_1 field has been turned on. Recall that the Larmor precessional frequency is given by $\omega_0 = \gamma B_0$. In Fig. 4-5B we have sketched what an observer on our merry-go-round would see if he were sitting atop and rotating with the B_1 field. Just as an observer on earth does not detect the earth's rotation because everything is moving at the same relative velocity, to our rotating magnetic observer all motion appears to have stopped. Interestingly, in our rotating system, because the precession of the magnetic moments has stopped ($\omega_0 = 0$), it is as though B_0 is absent ($\omega_0 = 0 = \gamma B_0$; $B_0 = 0$).

In this rotating system then, B_1 is the only field acting on the magnetization M, and M will begin to precess or rotate about B_1: $\omega_1 = \gamma B_1$ where, as noted before, $\gamma = 42.57$ MHz/T. The precession about B_1 will be slower than the precession about B_0 because B_1 is smaller. For a B_1 field of 24 G or 0.0024 T, the precessional frequency would be:

$$42.57\, \frac{\text{MHz}}{\text{T}} \times 0.0024\, \text{T} = 0.1\, \frac{\text{Megacycles}}{\text{sec}}$$

or $0.1 \times 10^{+6}$ cycles/sec. If a B_1 field of this magnitude (amplitude) were turned on for one μsec (10^{-6} sec), then M would have rotated about B_1 by 0.1 cycle ($0.1 \times 10^{+6} \times 10^{-6} = 0.1$), or 36°. If the field had been turned on for 2.5 μsec, then M would have rotated about B_1 by 0.25 ($\frac{1}{4}$) cycle. This is sketched in Fig. 4-5C, which also shows that M has been rotated about B_1 by 90°—this is a so-called 90° pulse of RF power. In Fig. 4-5D, a 180° pulse is sketched. This is achieved by allowing the B_1 field transmitter to be turned on for 5 μsec. By allowing the B_1 transmitter to be turned on for 10 μsec, M would have rotated one complete cycle (360°) and have ended where it started!

It should be emphasized that the pulse angle (or flip angle as it is sometimes called) depends on both the amplitude of the B_1 field and its duration. A weak B_1 field is often used in proton imaging for special purposes, and to attain the same flip angle with such a weak or "soft" B_1 pulse requires that it persists longer. For example, a B_1 field of 24 *milligauss* (0.0000024 T) would require a persistence time 1000 times longer to achieve the same flip angle as a strong or "hard" B_1 pulse of 24 G acting for microseconds.

An additional aspect of pulse angles worth emphasizing is that in the magnetic resonance literature, frequencies and pulse angles are often referred to in units of radians, rather than cycles. By definition, one cycle contains 2π radians. Consequently, as shown in Diagram 4-9, a 90° pulse is a $\pi/2$ pulse and a 180° pulse is a "π" pulse. Similarly, a proton resonance frequency of 42.57 MHz corresponds to an angular frequency of $42.57 \times 2\pi \times 10^{+6}$ radians/sec. Finally, we note that, by convention, when a rotating observer is used to illustrate the effect of magnetic fields on μ or M, the coordinate system on which he rotates is designated by primes (x',y',z').

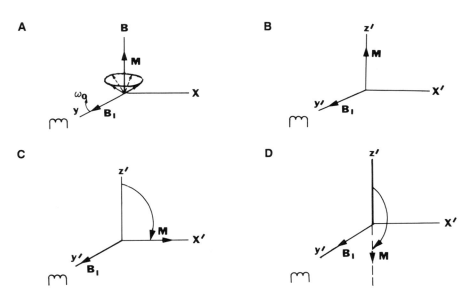

FIG. 4-5. Pulse angles to a rotating observer. **A:** Initial view of a stationary observer looking down the y axis—B_1 and μ's are rotating about B_0 at the Larmor frequency. **B:** Initial view of an observer rotating with the B_1 field—nothing is rotating, everything is stationary in a relative sense, and the B_0 field has disappeared! **C:** Initial view of an observer rotating with the B_1 field (0.0024 T), 2.5 μsec after turning the B_1 field on—a 90° pulse. **D:** Initial view of an observer rotating with the B_1 field (0.0024 T) 5 μsec after turning the B_1 field on—a 180° pulse.

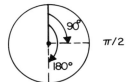

DIAGRAM 4-9. One cycle is 2π radians and a 180° pulse is a π pulse.

56 MAGNETIC RESONANCE WORKBOOK

QUESTIONS FOR SECTION 4.6

Complete the statements by circling a choice between the italicized options.

1. There *are* $\pi/2\pi$ radians in 360°.

2. The precession of M about B_1 is *slower/faster* than about B_0.

3. A 90° pulse corresponds to a $\pi/\pi/2$ pulse.

4. The longer the B_1 field is turned on, the *smaller/larger* is the pulse angle.

5. The stronger is the B_1 field of a pulse, the *larger/smaller* is the pulse angle.

6. A hard pulse is *longer/shorter* than an equivalent soft pulse.

7. On the merry-go-round, B_0 is *larger/smaller* than B_1 during the pulse.

4.7 Free Precession of M About B_0 After B_1 is Turned Off: Only Magnetization Precessing in the XY Plane Generates the Magnetic Resonance Signal

Fig. 4-5C provides the view by an observer rotating with the B_1 field immediately after it has rotated the sample magnetization by 90° or $\pi/2$ radians from the z' axis into the x'y' plane. If, after this 90° or $\pi/2$ pulse, the B_1 transmitter is turned off, what happens to the magnetization M? As shown in Fig. 4-6A, the magnetization, as viewed by a stationary observer looking down the y axis, executes a precession about the B_0 field at the Larmor frequency. The time-dependent voltage induced in the RF coil is sketched in Fig. 4-6B. This is the magnetic resonance signal.

It is important to emphasize that it is the magnetization component *precessing in the xy plane* that generates the magnetic resonance signal. For example, a π or 180° pulse was illustrated in Fig. 4-5D. Following this particular π pulse, the magnetization is along the $-z$ axis, has *no* component in the xy plane, and consequently will *not* generate a magnetic resonance signal. As we shall see in later sections, other types of π pulse can "create" xy magnetization and consequently have great utility in MRI. In this regard it is also important to note that it is not necessary to use a $\pi/2$ or 90° pulse to create xy magnetization. Fig. 4-6C shows the orientation of the magnetization immediately after the application of a 45° pulse. After the pulse, M has a component in the xy plane that will generate a signal;

however, because the component in the xy plane is smaller than the full magnetization created in the xy plane by π/2 pulse, the signal generated by the former will be weaker (have a smaller amplitude). Nonetheless, there are advantages that can be gained by the use of smaller flip angles (even less than 45°) in some of the fast imaging schemes.

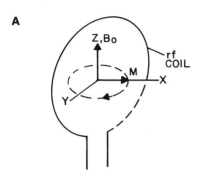

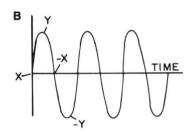

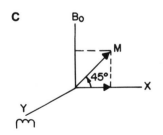

FIG. 4-6. Proton magnetic resonance signals are generated by free precession of magnetization in the xy plane. **A:** Free precession of M in the xy plane after the B_1 field along y has been turned off. M induces an AC current in a coil oriented in the yz plane. **B:** Time-dependent voltage induced in the RF coil by the free precession of M. Magnetization starts along +x (0 voltage), rotates to +y (maximum + voltage), continues to −x (0 voltage) and −y (maximum − voltage), and completes the cycles at +x. The rotation continues as long as M is in the xy plane. **C:** Orientation of the magnetization M immediately after a 45° pulse, which creates a component of magnetization in the xy plane.

Questions for Section 4.7 next page.

58 MAGNETIC RESONANCE WORKBOOK

QUESTIONS FOR SECTION 4.7

Complete the statements by circling a choice between the italicized options.

1. A 45° pulse creates *more/less* magnetization in the xy plane than does a 90° pulse.

2. The time-dependent voltage induced in the RF coil arises from *magnetization along the z axis/the component of M in the xy plane.*

5

Repetitive Generation of the Proton Magnetic Resonance Signal in Three Dimensions

5.1 Importance of Relaxation Processes and Initial Z Magnetization

In these next few sections, we introduce relaxation processes that restore magnetization along the z axis and destroy magnetization in the $x'y'$ plane after a B_1 pulse. An appreciation of these relaxation processes is central to understanding multiple pulse magnetic resonance imaging (MRI) methods and to evaluating the complex patterns of contrast in proton images.

In all clinically useful proton MRI procedures, the proton magnetic resonance signal for a given plane is generated, then there is a delay period, and the proton magnetic resonance signal for that plane is generated again. That procedure is repeated for the same plane a number of times for various reasons. One, as we have seen in Chapter 2, is to generate a sufficient number of phase-encoding steps to ensure the resolution required in the phase-encoding direction.

Each of the repetitions must create magnetization in the $x'y'$ plane to generate a nuclear magnetic resonance (NMR) signal. In turn, *this requires that magnetization preexist or be regenerated along the z axis so that a B_1 pulse can create magnetization in the $x'y'$ plane.* A corollary to this requirement is that somehow, between repetition of these pulses, magnetization disappears from the $x'y'$ plane. These requirements are illustrated graphically in Fig. 5-1A for the repetition of the two B_1 $\pi/2$ pulses. The first B_1 $\pi/2$ tilts the preexisting z magnetization M into the x'y' plane and generates a strong proton signal. After a delay, and without any processes that affect the magnetization in the x'y' plane, the next B_1 $\pi/2$ pulse rotates M to a position along the $-z'$ axis. No x'y' magnetization is created by this pulse and no proton NMR signal results. In fact, the second $\pi/2$ pulse removes the NMR signal.

In the actual tissue samples, something happens in the sample during the interval between the first and second $\pi/2$ pulses *to remove magneti-*

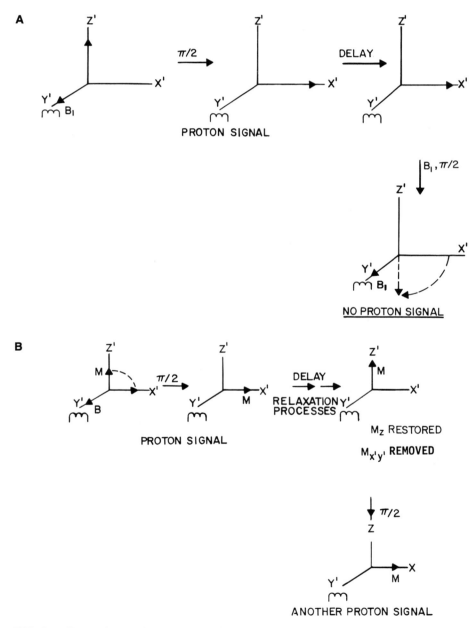

FIG. 5-1. Dependence of the proton signal on z magnetization. **A:** Depiction of the behavior of an initial proton magnetization under the influence of two B_1 $\pi/2$ pulses separated by a time delay during which nothing disturbs M in the x'y' plane after the first $\pi/2$ pulse. **B:** The pulse sequence of A, with relaxation included between $\pi/2$ pulses.

zation in the x'y' plane and restore magnetization along the z axis. These happenings, called relaxation processes, allow the second $\pi/2$ pulses now to "sample" magnetization along z and recreate M in the x'y' plane and generate another proton signal (Fig. 5-1B). In the next few sections, we will provide simple models for water proton relaxation processes in tissue samples.

QUESTIONS FOR SECTION 5.1

Complete the statements by circling a choice between the italicized options.

1. Relaxation processes can *create/destroy* magnetization in the x'y' plane and *restore/destroy* magnetization along the z axis.

   generate sufficient data to ensure the appropriate resolution in the phase-encoding direction.

2. Repetitive generation of magnetization in the x'y' plane during acquisition of data for the construction of a proton MRI is required because *the proton signal is strong/there is a need to*

3. Repetitive regeneration of magnetization in the x'y' plane by a $\pi/2$ pulse *requires that magnetization preexists or be regenerated along the z axis/is of little utility in MRI.*

5.2 Free Precession Does Not Last Forever: It Dies Out Because of Loss of Phase Coherence: Field Inhomogeneities

The voltage changes sketched in Fig. 4-6B define a free precession of M that lasts forever in the xy plane. The actual voltage change exhibited by a biological sample is illustrated in Fig. 5-2A in which the voltage and signal (Fig. 5-2B) die away in a damped oscillation characterized by an exponential decay ($\square\text{-}\text{-}\text{-}\text{-}$) with time. This damped oscillation and exponential decay are caused by the interaction of the xy magnetization with its surroundings in a manner that destroys the phase coherence created by the B_1 field. This occurs in several ways, the easiest of which to illustrate is the presence of inhomogeneities in the static field B_0.

As discussed in previous chapters, a highly homogeneous magnetic field means that all protons in the sample giving rise to the magnetic resonance signal experience exactly the same magnetic field strength and exactly the same precessional frequency. By exactly the same field strength, we mean to seven or eight decimal places—for a 1-T field, e.g., this means not 1.0

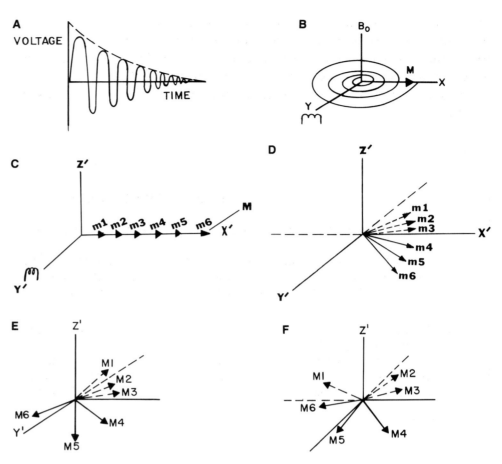

FIG. 5-2. Time dependence of the magnetization and the proton signal. **A:** Damped oscillation of the voltage with time induced by magnetization in the xy plane after a $\pi/2$ pulse on a tissue sample—the FID. **B:** Illustration of the time-dependent decay of xy magnetization that leads to the FID of signal. **C:** Magnetization M comprised of six components in an inhomogeneous magnetic field brought into phase coherence along the x' axis immediately after a B_1 $\pi/2$ pulse along y' at ω_0 (for B_0 = 1.0000000 T). **D:** Dephasing of the six Ms owing to field inhomogeneity 10 msec after the $\pi/2$ pulse. **E:** Continued dephasing of Ms owing to field inhomogeneity 20 msec after the $\pi/2$ pulse. **F:** Continued dephasing of Ms owing to field inhomogeneity 30 msec after the $\pi/2$ pulse.

T, but 1.0000000 T for all protons in the sample generating the magnetic resonance signal. This high degree of field homogeneity is difficult to achieve, but is necessary because the magnetogyric ratio of the proton is so large: 42,570,000 cycles/sec T (42.57 MHz/T). If two regions in the sample experience a magnetic field that differs by only 0.0000001 T, then the precessional frequencies of the protons in the two regions will differ by 42,579,000 × 0.0000001 = 4.257 cycles/sec. This means that in one second the protons in the minisculely higher field will have precessed by 4.257 cycles more than the protons in the B_0 field of exactly 1.0000000 T. Similarly, protons in a minisculely lower field of 0.9999999 T would have precessed 4.257 cycles less than protons in a B_0 field of 1.0000000 T. This is an important process for dephasing the xy magnetization!

Consider the highly simplified case of magnetization in the xy plane brought to phase coherence by a $\pi/2$ B_1 pulse. Six regions of the sample that are at slightly different magnetic fields contribute to the net magnetization M: M_1 (0.9999997 T), M_2 (0.9999998 T), M_3 (0.9999999 T), M_4

(1.0000001 T), M_5 (1.0000002 T), and M_6 (1.0000003 T). *Immediately* after the B_1 pulse the magnetization lies along the x' axis (Fig. 5-2C) and to an observer riding atop the y' axis at the Larmor frequency corresponding to a B_0 value of exactly 1.0000000 T, the magnetization from all six regions are in phase and comprise a stationary composite M. However, 10 msec after the $\pi/2$ pulse has been applied, M_4 will have traveled

$$4.257 \frac{\text{cycles}}{\text{sec}} \times 0.01 \text{ sec} = 0.04 \text{ cycles}$$

ahead of the observer in the B_0 of exactly 1.0000000 T. At 20 msec it will have traveled 0.08 cycles, and at 30 msec 0.12 cycles ahead. Similarly, at the same three time periods after the $\pi/2$ pulse, M_6 will have traversed 0.13 cycles

$$\left(42{,}570{,}000 \times 0.0000003 = 13 \frac{\text{cycles}}{\text{sec}} \times 0.01 \text{ sec} = 0.13 \right),$$

0.26 cycles, and 0.39 cycles ahead. Proceeding in a similar fashion we can prepare the following table of the number of cycles each of the M's gains (+) or loses (−) with respect to an observer precessing in a field exactly 1.0000000 T.

	Number of cycles gained (+) or lost (−)					
Time of observation	M_1	M_2	M_3	M_4	M_5	M_6
10 msec (0.01 sec)	−0.13	−0.08	−0.04	+0.04	+0.08	+0.13
20 msec	−0.26	−0.16	−0.08	+0.08	+0.16	+0.26
30 msec	−0.39	−0.24	−0.12	+0.12	+0.24	+0.39

These values are sketched in Figs. 5-2D through F. It is apparent from Fig. 5-2F that the magnetization components are almost completely dephased and that there is very little residual net magnetization M in the $x'y'$ plane 30 msec after the $\pi/2$ pulse (see Diagram 4-3). The proton signal will have nearly died away.

The loss of magnetization in the $x'y'$ plane by the loss of phase coherence is called the spin-spin relaxation process and is characterized by a time constant T_2 or T_2^* that we shall consider presently. However we should note two things here:

−The loss of phase coherence owing to field inhomogeneity is a nonrandom process (the same field inhomogeneities persist in the same volume for a long period of time); this nonrandom loss of phase coherence can be recovered with another appropriate B_1 pulse (Chapter 6).

−The loss of $x'y'$ magnetization by dephasing does not necessarily mean that this magnetization is recovered along the z' or z axis. Other processes are involved in the recovery of z magnetization and these are called spin-lattice relaxation processes characterized by a time constant T_1. However, spin-lattice relaxation *does* affect xy magnetization, as discussed in section 5.5.

QUESTIONS FOR SECTION 5.2

Select the one false statement:

1. The loss of phase coherence of magnetization in the xy plane is called spin-spin relaxation.

2. The loss of magnetization in the xy plane by the dephasing of proton spins is characterized by an exponential process with a time constant T_2.

3. A static magnetic field B_0 that is inhomogeneous will allow a free induction decay (FID) of magnetization in the xy plane to persist for a very long time.

4. The loss of phase coherence owing to field inhomogeneity is a nonrandom process.

5.3 Loss of Phase Coherence Owing to the Magnetization of the Tissue Sample Itself: Importance of Oscillations or Fluctuations of the Nuclear Magnetic Moments of Water in Tissue

In Section 5.2 we saw that the loss of phase coherence owing to magnetic field inhomogeneities acting over time leads to the loss of the magnetic resonance signal—implicit in the description is that the loss of phase coherence and signal is most rapid for large field inhomogeneities present for long times in the tissue sample. The inhomogeneous fields we considered were caused by the magnet or the interaction of the magnet with its surroundings as discussed in previous chapters. Conceptually, a similar dephasing effect can arise from the motion of nuclear magnets in the sample itself. Shown in Fig. 5-3 are two schematic water molecules [$H_2O(1)$ and $H_2O(2)$], each with one of their proton magnetic dipoles in close contact. For the time the μ_1 and μ_2 are close to one another in the orientation shown, the magnetic field of one adds to the external field provided by the magnet ($B_0 = 1.0000000$ T). The magnetic dipolar field can be quite large—for protons separated by $2A^0$, the field is 2 G (0.0002 T), representing a large temporary field inhomogeneity. For example, because of the effect of μ_2, μ_1 would process 8514 cycles/sec

$$\left(0.0002 \text{ T} \times 42.57 \times 10^{+6} \frac{\text{cycles}}{\text{sec}} = 8514 \right)$$

faster than a proton far away from a neighbor and experiencing an external field of exactly 1.0000000 T. This type of magnetic dipolar interaction could

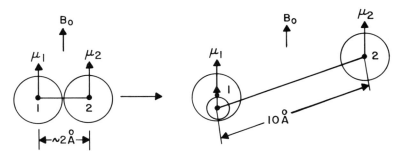

FIG. 5-3. Schematic of two water molecules, 1 and 2 initially in close contact such that two proton dipoles, μ_1 and μ_2, are within 2 A° (2 × 10^{-8} cm) of one another. The magnetic field created by μ_1 2A° from μ_2 is 2 G (0.0002 T). The water molecules stay in contact with one another for ~10^{-8} sec. When a collision with another water molecule separates them by 10 A° the field now created by μ_1 at μ_2 is only 0.016 G (0.00016 T).

result in such rapid dephasing of magnetization in the xy plane that it would be difficult to measure the rapidly decaying free induction signal. Fortunately it does not because collisions and rotations in the liquid water do not allow the two dipoles to maintain the close distance and their orientation for very long. In the example given in Fig. 5-3, the interaction persists for only 10^{-8} sec, leading to a dephasing by only 0.00008514 cycles

$$\left(8514 \frac{\text{cycles}}{\text{sec}} \times 10^{-8} \text{ sec}\right).$$

Nonetheless, so many such "close" collisions can take place in the 0.1 second or less during which we collect the signal (the FID), that the proton dipoles have time to become gradually dephased by this process.

The magnetic dipolar interactions just described are intermolecular—they occur *between* water molecules. Fluctuating *intramolecular* dipolar fields also can cause loss of phase coherence of the proton dipoles. The oxygen atom of the water molecule is bonded to *two protons that are in constant, rapid vibrational* [∧] *and rotational* [∧] *motion*. These intramolecular motions of one proton dipole with respect to the other produce strong oscillating magnetic fields at the other dipole with a wide range of persistence times (10^{-4}–10^{-12} sec) that effectively destroy phase coherence.

In these simple pictures, we have oversimplified greatly the complex motions and magnetic dipolar interactions that occur in a liquid such as water. For example, some types of contacts persist for as long as 10^{-3} sec (causing, e.g., a "dephasing" in the model of Fig. 5-3 of 8.514 cycles). A complete description of dephasing of the water protons by these magnetic dipolar interactions requires an analysis of the types, distances, and persistence (or frequency of change) of near and "far" interactions. For our purposes it is sufficient to realize that the process is an effective one for dephasing the water proton dipoles. In this context it should be noted that for the pure liquid water, it takes approximately 30 sec for the water dipoles to dephase *completely* after a $\pi/2$ pulse at a $B_0 \geq 0.50000$ T.

QUESTIONS FOR SECTION 5.3

Select the one false statement:

1. The strength of the magnetic dipolar interactions of the protons on two different water molecules increases as the water molecules get closer to each other.

2. The shorter the period of time that two proton magnetic dipoles are in close contact, the more quickly they lose phase coherence owing to magnetic dipolar interactions.

3. A highly homogeneous magnetic field means that all protons in the sample giving rise to the magnetic resonance signal experience exactly the same magnetic field strength and exactly the same precessional frequency.

4. Even in a perfectly homogeneous magnetic field, the FID of tissue water protons would not last forever because of dephasing caused by magnetic dipolar interactions in the tissue.

5.4 Loss of Phase Coherence Owing to Tissue Magnetization: Macromolecules in the Water

When large molecules such as lipids or proteins are present in aqueous solutions or dispersions, the time required for a complete dephasing of the *water* proton dipoles after a $\pi/2$ B_1 pulse can be reduced by a factor of *10 or more* compared to pure water, depending on the concentration, size, and type of molecule. How does this more efficient dephasing (signal loss) occur? Segments of the molecule carry large, effective magnetic moments and these segments exhibit relatively slow motions that allow relatively long persistence times for the "contact" with the net magnetization of the water protons.

Fig. 5-4A shows the structure of a short segment of a protein, which is a large macromolecule composed of amino acid units. The segment can exhibit a net magnetic moment in a B_0 field that is composed of the sum of the individual moments of the CH, NH, and OH proton dipoles. This net effective magnetic moment depends on the nature of the motion of the molecule and its segments, fast motions generally leading to a reduction of the net effective magnetic moment through an averaging (cancellation) of the sum of the individual CH, NH, and OH proton magnetic moments. Because of mechanical considerations, smaller molecules and segments move (rotate and translate) faster than larger molecules and segments. For the segment of the macromolecule shown schematically in Fig. 5-4B, this moment is larger (say, a factor of 10 or more) than the individual proton magnetic moments of the water proton dipoles and the field at the proton dipole would be up to 20 G (0.002 T) more than the B_0 field. Because of the "contact" between ⇑ and O, the water proton dipoles would precess up to 85,140 cycles/sec faster than a water proton far away from the protein and experiencing only the external B_0 field. This is an effective process for dephasing the magnetization M of the water proton dipoles after a $\pi/2$ B_1 pulse, because: (a) there is a large variety of "contact distances (and effective dipolar fields) between macromolecular segments and water molecules, (b) macromolecules move (translate and rotate) much more slowly than small water molecules, and (c) water molecules "stick" (actually bind) to proteins for a time longer than they bind to each other. Thus the interaction depicted in Fig. 5-4B might persist for 10^{-6} sec or longer before a collision or rotation caused a large separation of O and ⇑. In that time period the amount that the water proton becomes dephased would be 0.0805 cycles (85,140 cycles/sec × 0.000001 sec). For a different contact that persisted for 10^{-5} to 10^{-4} sec, the phase shift of a water proton might be as large as 0.8 to 8 cycles.

In summary, the macromolecule is a much more effective agent for dephasing water proton dipoles than are water protons themselves because large net magnetic moments can be induced in segments of macromolecules

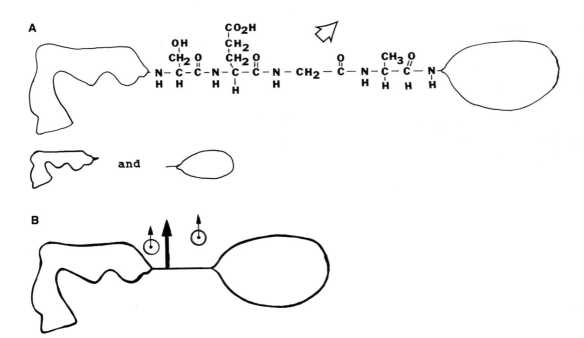

FIG. 5-4. Interaction of water proton dipoles with proteins. **A:** Structure of a short segment of a protein showing the amino acids that comprise it. The segment shown has an approximate "molecular weight" of 360. The protein has other large amino acid chain segments, denoted at the bottom portion of this figure, and has a molecular weight as large as 50,000–350,000 Dalton. Depending on the exact structure of the segment and the protein, the segment can exhibit in a static magnetic field a net magnetic moment comprised of the individual moments μ of the NH, CH, and OH protons. **B:** Water molecules with their proton dipoles, O oriented along the protein segment magnetic moment, ⇑. ⇑ is a factor of 10 larger than O. For a separation of 2A° the field at O due ⇑ is 20 G or .002 T.

68 MAGNETIC RESONANCE WORKBOOK

by the B_0 field, and the contact between the induced magnetization and the water proton dipole persists for a longer period of time. Again this is a very simple *conceptual* model and a detailed accounting of water proton dephasing in protein solutions requires a more complete assessment of induced magnetization of segments, stickiness of water (a controversial subject), types of motion possible and their rates, and protein types and concentrations.

Finally we note that the dephasing of the proton dipoles by fluctuating internal fields is a random irreversible process, unlike the dephasing caused by persistent magnetic field inhomogeneities. In the random process, one collision with an internal field might shift the water proton phase by a tenth of a cycle, the next by a hundredth, the next by 10 cycles, and so on. Because many such collisions occur during the free precession of M, the dephasing brought about by random fluctuating fields cannot be refocused by B_1 pulses, in contrast to the situation with magnetic field inhomogeneities.

QUESTIONS FOR SECTION 5.4

Select the one true statement:

1. Macromolecules dissolved in water generally increase the water proton spin-spin relaxation times.

2. The longer T_2 is, the faster the magnetization in the xy plane dephases.

3. The dephasing of magnetization in the xy plane always leads to recovery of magnetization along the z axis.

4. The effectiveness of T_2 relaxation of water protons by a dissolved macromolecule depends both on the strength of the water-protein magnetic dipolar interaction and its persistence time.

5. A magnetic dipolar interaction that shifts the water proton resonance frequency by 1000 Hz and persists for 1 msec will shift the phase of the water proton resonance by 100 cycles.

5.5 The Recovery of Magnetization Along the Z Axis: General Aspects of Spin-Lattice Relaxation

The processes we have described so far are effective in causing loss of signal in the $x'y'$ plane, but they do not necessarily lead to *recovery* of magnetization along the z axis. As noted before, spin-lattice relaxation (or

T_1) processes are responsible for the recovery of z magnetization, and this occurs efficiently in tissue samples at the same rate or somewhat more slowly than magnetization, which is *lost* or *dephased* in the x'y' plane.

When the proton magnetization is supplied a $\pi/2$ pulse by a B_1 field and rotated into the x'y' plane, the magnetization (or spin system) "heats up" (Fig. 5-5). Conversely, when spin-lattice relaxation processes allow rotation of M from the xy plane back to alignment with B_0 along the z axis, M releases energy to the lattice, thereby heating it up. The magnetic energy released by M is converted to increased rates of rotation and collision of segments of the lattice—its temperature rises with continued cycling of M from alignment with B_0 to rotation into the xy plane, and reorientation along B_0. This is a true relaxation process, because M relaxes from a state of high energy (in the xy plane) to a state of low energy (aligned along z and B_0).

All systems tend to flow (relax) from a state of high energy to the lowest energy state accessible and, in our spin system, T_1 relaxation is the path by which this occurs. A car in neutral gear near the top of a hill (high energy state) will roll downhill (low energy state) if the brake is released. There is a natural brake in our spin system that makes spontaneous emission of the relatively low magnetic energy of M in the xy plane to the thermal "bath" of the lattice an extremely slow process. The T_1 path circumvents the brake through magnetic dipolar interactions between M and the lattice. The T_1 process depends on the fluctuations of induced magnetization in the sample (lattice) but, unlike the case for T_2 relaxation, the more rapid fluctuations lead to effective spin-lattice relaxation. Indeed, those fluctuations in the lattice that occur at the Larmor frequency (ω_0) are most effective.

We can use a simplified conceptual model to rationalize this. Consider the small hydrogen bonded segment of water sketched in Diagram 5-1. Segments such as these in the water "lattice" are in constant rotational, vibrational, and translational motion, which leads to rapid fluctuation of the segmental induced magnetization ⇒ (dipolar field). These fluctuations range in frequency from 10^{+12} sec^{-1} to 10^{+6} sec^{-1} or lower. At some

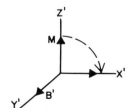

FIG. 5-5. Energy is absorbed and then released in the cycling of the magnetization from the z axis to the xy plane and back again. A: The B_1 field rotating at ω_0 twists M into the x'y' plane in a $\pi/2$ pulse, thereby raising its energy. The energy is supplied by the B_1 transmitter and the spin system (magnetic dipoles comprising M) "heats up".

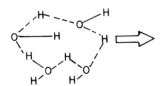

DIAGRAM 5-1. Small hydrogen bonded segment of a water "lattice" showing a net induced magnetization.

location in the lattice we can conceive a dipolar field rotating at ω_0 in the configuration depicted in Fig. 5-6. This configuration provides a means to visualize how M as a "hot" spin system in the x'y' plane can transfer that spin energy to the dipolar field in the lattice as M relaxes back to the low energy alignment as a "cool" spin system along z and B_0. The efficient exchange of energy between M and the lattice depends on the strength of the dipolar field with frequency components that maintain their fluctuations at ω_0.

Of course this process is highly idealized. The "flickering clusters" of the water lattice shown in Diagram 5-1 have a wide distribution of rotation frequencies, and the frequency of rotation of a particular cluster will be accelerated or slowed down by frequent collisions with other water molecules. Consequently, the restoration of M along z is a stepwise process in which ⇑ provided by a few flickering clusters acting for a short period of time allows the rotation of M by a small amount, the process being interrupted by collisions and subsequently continued by another set of "flickering clusters" (Diagram 5-2). Note that this spin-lattice relaxation process also removes magnetization from the xy plane—in this process spin-spin and spin-lattice relaxation occur together.

As with T_2 relaxation, the presence of proteins in aqueous solution can cause large reductions in the *water* proton T_1, depending on the size, shape, and composition of the protein. We can attribute the increased efficiency of water proton spin-lattice relaxation processes in these protein solutions to the presence of larger dipolar fields in protein segments that are fluctuating at the Larmor frequency (ω_0). In this context, note that we have used the terms fluctuation and rotations interchangeably in this discussion. In our simple models of relaxation, we have depicted the dipolar fields as *rotating* at ω_0. But, as we have shown in Section 4.4, a linearly fluctuating field that might arise, e.g., from a wagging translational motion of a protein segment (or water cluster) can be represented by a rotating field.

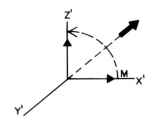

FIG. 5-6. Water proton magnetization M is in the x'y' plane immediately after A $\pi/2$ B_1 pulse applied along the y' axis. The B field has been turned off. A segment of the water lattice with a net magnetization ⇒ is rotating at precisely the Larmor frequency of M. To an observer rotating on y' at the Larmor frequency, M and ⇒ appear to be stationary. This configuration allows energy exchange between M and the dipolar field, and clockwise rotation of M about ⇒ will be observed, allowing the return of M to alignment along Z' (B_0) in a random stepwise fashion.

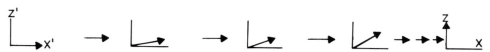

DIAGRAM 5-2. Multistep processes govern the rate of recovery of z magnetization by spin-lattice relaxation. Note that this spin-lattice relaxation process also removes magnetization from the x'y' plane. In this process spin-spin and spin-lattice relaxation occur together.

QUESTIONS FOR SECTION 5.5

Select the two true statements:

1. Recovery of magnetization along the z axis after a $\pi/2$ pulse does not necessarily result in loss of magnetization from the xy plane.

2. The closer the rate of rotation of a magnetized segment of an aqueous protein is to the proton Larmor frequency, the less effective the segment is in allowing T_1 relaxation of water protons.

3. Spin-lattice relaxation is a random process.

4. Water molecules rotate more slowly than macromolecules in aqueous solution.

5. Aqueous protein solutions generally have longer water proton spin-lattice relaxation times than does pure water at the same temperature.

6. Spin-lattice relaxation of magnetization literally heats up the lattice.

7. When a B_1 pulse tilts the magnetization away from the z axis by a $\pi/2$ angle, energy is transferred from the proton dipoles to the RF coil.

8. When the magnetization relaxes from the xy plane back to the z axis, it absorbs energy from the lattice.

5.6 Spin-Lattice and Spin-Spin Relaxation Processes are Exponential Processes Characterized by Different Time Dependencies

We have already seen that spin-spin relaxation (Sections 5.2 and 5.3) can occur by a process completely independent of spin-lattice relaxation. This spin-spin relaxation in biological tissue usually occurs somewhat more quickly than spin-lattice relaxation. Both processes we have described *are exponential processes*—the magnetization in the x'y' plane starts out large and gets smaller because of collisions, rotations, and magnetic field inhomogeneities and, as the x'y' magnetization gets smaller, it becomes more difficult to reduce the smaller magnetization remaining.

The exponential process for spin-spin relaxation is sketched in Fig. 5-7—in it the magnetization initially falls off (decays) quickly with time and then decays more slowly at later times. The time, t = 0 is the time immediately after the application of the B_1 $\pi/2$ pulse when the xy magnetization is at the maximum value, $M_{xy}(0)$. At any other time the magnetization, $M_{xy}(t)$ is less owing to spin-spin relaxation $M_{xy}(t) = M_{xy}(0)(e^{-t/T_2})$. The exponential part of the process is summarized in the

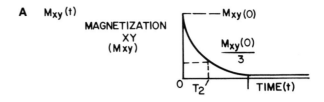
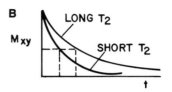
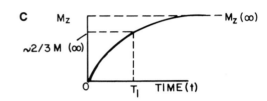

FIG. 5-7. The T_1 and T_2 processes exhibit an exponential time dependence. **A:** Exponential decay of xy or x'y' magnetization with time. This also represents loss of proton magnetic resonance signal. The loss of magnetization (M_{xy}) follows the equation $M_{xy}(t) = M_{xy}(0)e^{-t/T_2}$. **B:** Exponential decay of M_{xy} for a tissue with rapid (short T_2) and slow (long T_2) spin-spin relaxation. **C:** Exponential growth of M_z with time. The growth of z magnetization follows the equation $M_z(t) = M_z(\infty)(1 - e^{-t/T_1})$.

exponential term, e^{-t/T_2} where T_2 is the spin-spin relaxation time characteristic of the tissue being studied. It is the time, $t = T_2$ for which $e^{-T_2/T_2} = e^{-1} = 0.37$, and

$$M_{xy}(t) = M_{xy}(0)(0.37) = 0.37\, M_{xy}(0) = \sim\tfrac{1}{3}\, M_{xy}(0),$$

or the time when the magnetization has decayed to $\sim\tfrac{1}{3}$ its initial value. Tissues with rapid spin-spin relaxation have short T_2 values; tissues with slow spin-spin relaxation have long T_2 values (Fig. 5-7B). Tissues generally have T_2 values in the range of 0.02 to 0.2 sec (20 msec to 200 msec). These depend only slightly on the strength of the B_0 field, a subject to be discussed later.

Similarly, spin-lattice relaxation follows an exponential process but in this case we plot the recovery (or gain) of magnetization along the z or z' axis (Fig. 5-7C). The time, $t = 0$, is the time immediately after the application of the B_1 $\pi/2$ pulse when the magnetization along z is 0, $M_z = 0$. At very long times, $t = \infty$, the magnetization along z is back almost exactly to its maximum value (99.99999999999...% of it) $M_z(\infty)$. The exponential part of the process is now contained in the term, $1 - e^{-t/T_1}$, where T_1 is the spin-lattice relaxation time during which the magnetization has recovered to $\tfrac{2}{3}$ its maximum value:

$$M_z(T_1) = M_z(\infty)(1 - e^{-T_1/T_1}) = M_z(\infty)(1-0.37) = 0.63\, M_z(\infty) \simeq \tfrac{2}{3} M_z(\infty).$$

Again, tissues with rapid spin-lattice relaxation have short values of T_1. The T_1 values of tissue vary from 0.2 to 1.2 sec, depending on the strength of the static magnetic field B_0. A fact of nature of considerable importance in MRI is that T_2 is equal to or less than T_1—spin-spin relaxation occurs as fast as or faster than spin-lattice relaxation. It is found that T_2 generally is less than T_1.

QUESTIONS FOR SECTION 5.6

Select the two true statements:

1. The recovery of z magnetization by spin-lattice relaxation is an exponential process in which the initial stages of recovery are slower than the late stages.

2. The loss of magnetization in the xy plane by spin-spin relaxation is an exponential process in which the initial stages of the loss occur more quickly than the later stages.

3. T_2 is an intrinsic property of tissue and it is the time when the magnetization $M_{xy}(0)$ has decayed to $\sim \frac{1}{3}$.

4. Tissue T_2 is always larger than or equal to tissue T_1.

5. A short tissue T_1 indicates a slow spin-lattice relaxation process.

6. The proton T_1 and T_2 values of water solutions usually can be lengthened by adding macromolecules.

6

The Influences of T_1 and T_2 on Imaging Time and Image Intensity and Contrast

6.1 T_1 and the Repetition Time, T_R

As discussed in Chapter 2, the basic steps involved in the construction of the simple proton images include: (a) imposition of a gradient on the static field B_0 such that a specific volume in the subject has all protons precessing at a specific frequency (e.g., ω_1 different from all other resonance frequencies of the subject in the B_0 field along its gradient), (b) excitation of all protons in the volume selected with a frequency specific (ω_1) pulse of B_1 irradiation—in our three-dimensional (3D) model, this corresponds to rotation of the magnetization in the selected volume from alignment with z into the $x'y'$ plane, (c) with the volume selective gradient off and the B_1 field off, another gradient at right angles to the first is turned on for a short time to encode the phase of the spins as a function of position, and (d) a frequency-encoding gradient is turned on at right angles to the first two gradients while the signal is being collected, 128, 256, or 512 data points in the frequency-encoding direction being collected. This latter defines resolution in the frequency direction. To obtain an equivalent resolution in the phase direction, 128, 256, or 512 phase-encoding steps would need to be used. *Each phase-encoding step requires repeating process (a) through (d) above.* Thus, for a resolution of 256 points in the phase-encoding direction, (a) through (d) would be repeated 256 times with the amplitude of the phase-encoding gradient being changed each time.

This requirement of individual phase-encoding steps puts severe constraints on the minimum time required to collect the imaging data because *the time elapsed, T_R between the repetition of steps (a) through (d) must be long enough to allow recovery of z magnetization.* Approximately 99% of the z magnetization recovers if a time interval $T_R = 5T_1$ is allowed to elapse before repeating the phase-encoding cycle. For a tissue having a $T_1 = 1$ sec, this means that for a resolution of 256 points over the volume of interest it would require at least 1280 sec (256 × 1 × 5) to obtain the phase-encoding information. For a resolution of 516 points, 2560 seconds (~43 min) would be required!

Obviously great lengths are taken to devise imaging schemes that reduce the time required for obtaining the phase-encoding data. A simple time-saving modification would be to reduce T_R—if $T_R = T_1$ were chosen, we would save a factor of 5 in time. As in all other time-saving schemes we will discuss later, there are trade-offs. In this case, one of the trade-offs would be a loss in signal intensity—only the first B_1 pulse would sample the full magnetization along the z axis, $M_z(\infty)$. In the repetition time T_R after this first B_1 pulse, only $\frac{2}{3} M_z(\infty)$ would have recovered along the z axis and this would be the magnetization sampled by the second B_1 pulse. The second pulse would provide only $\frac{2}{3}$ the signal that the first provided (Fig. 6-1). There are other technical difficulties with this imaging scheme that we will take up in subsequent texts.

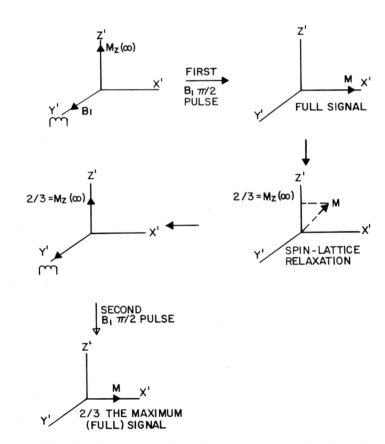

FIG. 6-1. Two consecutive $\pi/2$ pulses separated by $T_R = T_1$. The second pulse generates $\frac{2}{3}$ the signal intensity of the first.

QUESTIONS FOR SECTION 6.1

Select the two true statements:

1. As T_R is increased, the imaging time is decreased.

2. As T_R is decreased, the intensity in a proton image usually increases.

3. The imaging time increases as the number of phase-encoding steps increases.

4. The spin-lattice relaxation time is an important factor to consider in the selection of T_R.

5. If it requires 10 min to obtain a resolution of 256 phase-encoding points in an image, then 20 min would be required to obtain a resolution of 128 phase-encoding points.

6.2 The Use of T_R to Increase the Difference in Signal Intensity Between Tissue Structures Having Different T_1 Values: T_1 Weighted (Attenuated) Contrast

Consider the two tissue sample compartments sketched in Fig. 6-2. In this exaggerated example, the compartments are of the same size, contain the same amount of water, but have much different spin-lattice relaxation times because tissue compartment 1 has elevated levels of protein that enhance spin-lattice relaxation. By now we know that the signal intensity (S) is proportional to $M_z(\infty)$. $M_z(\infty)$, in turn, is proportional to the amount of water (N) in the volume being imaged:

$$S \propto M_z(\infty) \propto N.$$

What is the signal intensity in the image of compartment 1 relative to compartment 2? It depends on the imaging method used! If we used a method consisting of a simple B_1 $\pi/2$ pulse to generate the signal and waited $T_R = 5T_1$ (where T_1 is the value for compartment 2) to repeat the pulse for the acquisition of signals for each of the phase-encoding steps, then both compartments would have the *same signal intensity*. Both have the same amount of water and each B_1 pulse would sample the same $M_z(\infty)$, which would have fully recovered along the z axis after each pulse. This situation is sketched in Fig. 6-2B.

If, however, we select a repetition time that is 5 times the T_1 value for compartment 1, then the image intensity will be greater for compartment 1 because after the repetitive $\pi/2$ B_1 pulses the magnetization M_z will fully recover for compartment 1 but not for the more slowly relaxing compartment 2. This situation is sketched in Fig. 6-2C. The relative values of the signal intensities can be approximated from the appropriate exponential equations, noting that $M_z(\infty)$ for compartments 1 and 2 are equal:

$$\text{Signal (compartment 1)} = M_z(\infty)(1-e^{-0.75/0.15})$$
$$= M_z(\infty)(1-0.01)$$
$$= 0.99\ M_z(\infty)$$
$$\text{Signal (compartment 2)} = M_z(\infty)(1-e^{-0.75/0.5})$$
$$= M_z(\infty)(1-0.2)$$
$$= 0.8\ M_z(\infty).$$

Thus the signal from compartment 2 will be approximately 20% less than that from compartment 1. Compartment 1 will be appreciably brighter in the image. This T_1 weighting (or, more correctly, attenuation) can be further enhanced by picking an even shorter T_R value. But remember, the price we pay is loss of signal intensity in both compartments!

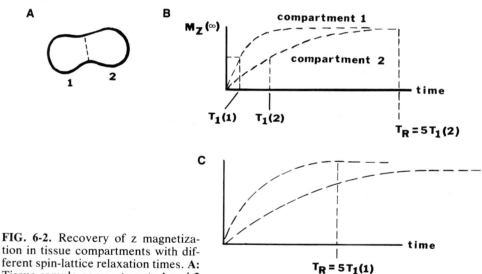

FIG. 6-2. Recovery of z magnetization in tissue compartments with different spin-lattice relaxation times. **A:** Tissue sample compartments 1 and 2 of the same size containing the same amount of water. Compartment 1 is diseased tissue containing twice the protein concentration of the normal tissue in compartment 2. The spin-lattice relaxation time of water in compartment 1 is 0.15 sec, whereas the T_1 of water in normal compartment 2 is 0.50 sec. **B:** Magnetization in both compartments fully recovers after repetitive B_1 $\pi/2$ pulses if T_R is chosen to be 5× the longer of the T_1 values of the compartments [5 × $T_1(2)$]. **C:** Magnetization is fully recovered only in compartment 1 after repetitive $\pi/2B_1$ pulses if T_R is chosen to be the shorter of the T_1 values of the compartments [$T_R = 5T_1(1)$].

QUESTIONS FOR SECTION 6.2

Select the two true statements:

1. If two tissue compartments have the same proton density, then each necessarily must have the same signal intensity in a proton magnetic resonance image (MRI).

2. Two tissue compartments have equal proton densities, but one has a T_1 of 1000 msec and the other has a T_1 of 500 msec; therefore, the contrast in proton MRIs of the two compartments will be greater at a $T_R = 5000$ msec than at $T_R = 500$ msec.

3. $e^{-5/2}$ is a smaller number than $e^{-2/5}$.

4. $(1-e^{-5/2})$ is a larger number than $(1-e^{-2/5})$.

5. Two tissue compartments have equal proton densities and equal T_1 values; therefore, contrast between the two compartments in proton images is best increased by choosing very short T_R values.

6. T_1 enhancement of contrast in proton MRI can be accomplished without paying the price of the reduction of signal intensity somewhere in the image.

6.3 Magnetization in the XY Plane Lost by Field Inhomogeneity Dephasing Can Be Recovered with a π (180°) Pulse: Spin Echoes and T_E

As we have noted earlier, loss of magnetization in the xy plane because of magnetic field inhomogeneities is not a random process—the inhomogeneities persist for a long time and are remembered by the spin system. This allows the magnetization to be refocused by an appropriate B_1 pulse, a π or 180° pulse. The effect of a simple π pulse is shown in Fig. 6-3A. Now consider the six magnetization components of Fig. 5-2E, which are dephasing because of inhomogeneities in the static magnetic field B_0. Recall that to our observer riding atop the y' axis at the Larmor frequency, M_6 is precessing more quickly and M_1 is precessing more slowly. As a consequence, in 20 msec M_6 has gained 0.26 cycles of phase compared to the observer. If a π pulse is applied to this system along y', then the magnetization components will now be aligned, as shown in Fig. 6-3B. After the π pulse, M_6 is still precessing more quickly and M_1 is still precessing more slowly than the observer along y'. What happens 20 msec after the π pulse? To our observer riding along y', M_6 will appear to have gained 0.26 cycles of phase and be aligned along x', while M_1 will appear to have lost 0.26 cycles of phase and will also be aligned along the x' axis!

Similarly M_2, M_3, M_4, and M_5 will be aligned, creating a strong proton magnetic resonance signal. This signal is called a "spin echo". Note that the spin echo does not contain any components that have been irreversibly dephased because of the *random* fluctuating fields present within the sample. Consequently the "spin echo" signal will be smaller than the free induction decay (FID) immediately after a $\pi/2$ pulse. The 20-msec delay after the $\pi/2$ pulse after which the π pulse is applied, is called the "time to echo" or the echo evolution time, T_E. The longer the T_E, the smaller the FID of the spin echo signal because more time will have been allowed for irreversible dephasing owing to random fields within the sample.

We call the spin-spin relaxation time owing to the intrinsic random fluctuating fields within the sample the intrinsic or true T_2 value. The intrinsic T_2 values of tissue vary widely depending on the tissue properties and provide an additional means of enhancing contrast in proton MRIs.

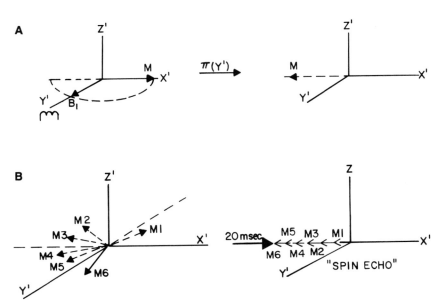

FIG. 6-3. Effect of π pulses on magnetization already in the x'y' plane. **A:** If immediately after a $\pi/2$ pulse that tilts M from z to alignment along x', a π (180°) pulse is applied along y', then M becomes aligned along the $-x'$ axis. **B:** The alignment of the magnetization components of FIG. 5-2E after a π pulse applied along the y' axis—all components are rotated 180° about the y' axis. To an observer riding along the y' axis 20 msec later, all the magnetization components become realigned along the $-x'$ axis, creating a strong magnetic resonance signal called a "spin echo".

QUESTIONS FOR SECTION 6.3

Select the one true statement:

1. Magnetization dephased by random processes can be refocused with a π pulse.

2. The intensity of a tissue proton spin echo obtained after $2T_E = 40$ msec should be larger than the intensity of one obtained after $2T_E = 80$ msec.

3. Intrinsic T_2 values of tissue are not important in the selection of $2T_E$ in proton imaging schemes.

4. The discussion in Section 6.3 involves the pulse sequence $\pi/2$, wait, π, wait, acquire FID. The pulse sequence π, wait, $\pi/2$, wait, acquire FID will provide the same information.

6.4 The Use of $2T_E$ to Increase the Difference in Signal Intensity Between Tissue Structures Having Different Intrinsic T_2 Values: T_2 Weighted (Attenuated) Contrast

Up to now, we have considered obtaining the magnetic resonance signal by recording the FID immediately after the application of a B_1 $\pi/2$ pulse, which tips the z magnetization into the xy plane. We now know we have the option of waiting a time T_E, applying an additional π pulse, and then recording the spin echo FID after waiting an additional time T_E for the magnetization to refocus. The total time that will have elapsed between applying the $\pi/2$ pulse and recording the signal is $2T_E$, and this is a time period, $t = 2T_E$, during which the magnetization can irreversibly decay by the intrinsic T_2 spin-spin relaxation process according to the equation used before:

$$M_{xy}(t) = M_{xy}(0)e^{-t/T_2}.$$

By varying this echo evolution time, $2T_E$, we can enhance the contrast (difference in image intensity) between two adjacent tissue compartments that have the same proton concentration and nearly identical T_1 values, but different T_2 values.

Consider again our simple two compartment model (Fig. 6-4A). In this model, the diseased tissue in compartment 1 has the same water proton concentration (density) as compartment 2, which is the same size. The protein content in 1 is somewhat elevated relative to 2, but the T_1 spin-lattice relaxation times of water in the two compartments are nearly iden-

FIG. 6-4. Decay of magnetization in the xy plane for tissue compartments with different T_2 values. **A:** Two tissue compartments of the same size containing the same water proton concentration. Diseased tissue of Compartment 1 has a slightly elevated protein concentration which does not affect T_1 but does lower the intrinsic T_2 of water in Compartment 1 (T_2 = 80 msec) compared to that in Compartment 2 (T_2 = 120 msec). **B:** The decay of magnetization, M_{xy}, for two compartments of the same size having identical water concentrations but different values of the intrinsic spin-spin relaxation times. By acquiring the FID of the spin echo after a pulse sequence, $\pi/2$, T_E, π, T_E, acquire, more signal is acquired from Compartment 2, which has the longer spin-spin relaxation time.

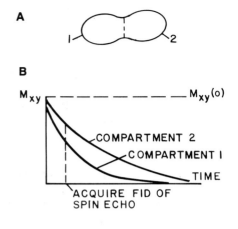

tical. However, as is often the case, the protein content affects the intrinsic T_2 much more than it does T_1 and the water in compartment 1 has a T_2 of 80 msec, whereas that in normal compartment 2 has a T_2 of 120 msec. The proton intensity for the two compartments in images obtained by obtaining the FID immediately after a $\pi/2$ pulse would be the same with and without T_1 enhancement (attenuation). However, if we employed the pulse sequence $\pi/2$, T_E, π, T_E, acquire FID; wait $5T_1$; repeat, then the signal intensities for the two compartments *would* differ by an amount dependent on T_E (Fig. 6-4B). For example, for T_E = 20 msec ($2T_E$ = 40 msec),

$$\text{Signal (compartment 1)} = M_{xy}(0)e^{-40/80}$$
$$= M_{xy}(0)\, 0.60$$
$$= 0.60\, M_{xy}(0)$$
$$\text{Signal (compartment 2)} = M_{xy}(0)e^{-40/120}$$
$$= M_{xy}(0)\, 0.75$$
$$= 0.75\, M_{xy}(0).$$

The signal intensities in the two compartments would be different by more than 20%. If, on the other hand, we waited for an echo evolution time of 40 msec ($2T_E$ = 80 msec) then the signal intensities in the two compartments would differ by more than 30%.

$$\text{Signal (1)} = M_{xy}(0)e^{-80/80} = 0.37\, M_{xy}(0)$$
$$\text{Signal (2)} = M_{xy}(0)e^{-80/120} = 0.50\, M_{xy}(0).$$

Note, however, that by waiting the additional time to improve contrast, we have lost signal from both compartments: signal from 1 at 80 msec is only 37% and signal 2 is only 50% of that attainable [$M_{xy}(0)$] without *any* delay in collecting the FID. This is a common theme in proton MRI: *what is done to improve contrast usually decreases the signal throughout the image.*

6.5 Most Proton Images Obtained Using Spin Echo Techniques are Both T_1 and T_2 Weighted (Attenuated): A Practical Consequence is That a Reduction in Tissue T_1 Causes a Relative Increase in Image Intensity, But a Reduction in Tissue Intrinsic T_2 Causes a Relative Decrease in Image Intensity

A common simplified spin echo pulse sequence is shown in Fig. 6-5. As in the simple model discussed in Chapter 2, a frequency selective $\pi/2 B_1$ pulse rotates the magnetization of the protons from the z axis in a plane selected by a field gradient G_z. The protons now along x' in the plane selected are precessing in phase at the Larmor frequency. B_1 and G_z are turned off and a phase-encoding gradient is turned on to encode spatially the resonances along the G phase direction and then it is turned off. Then the xy magnetization of the plane selected is allowed to dephase naturally for a period T_E after which a π pulse is applied. Near a time $2T_E$, the magnetization that has been dephased by field inhomogeneities begins to refocus, a frequency-encoding gradient is turned on, and the FID of the spin echo is recorded. Note that during the period $2T_E$ irreversible dephasing occurs owing to intrinsic T_2 relaxation, and that portion of the spin echo signal is lost. After a period T_R the whole process is repeated to obtain the full phase-encoding information in 128, 256, or 512 steps, depending on the resolution necessary.

The dependence of the signal intensity on T_R, T_E, T_1, and T_2 (intrinsic), and the proton density or concentration N (note that N is proportional to $M_{xy}(0)$ and $M_z(\infty)$) is given by:

$$\text{Signal} \propto N(1 - e^{-T_R/T_1})e^{-2T_E/T_2}.$$

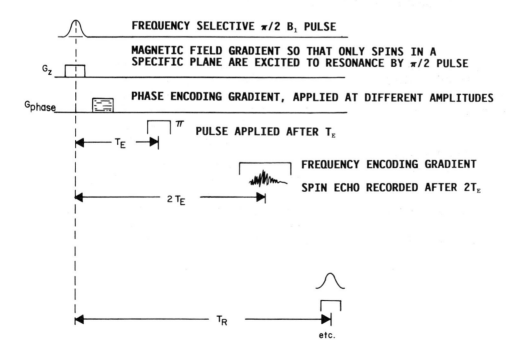

FIG. 6-5. Timing diagram for a simplified spin echo imaging sequence.

84 Magnetic Resonance Workbook

The dependence of the signal intensity from two compartments of equal size and water concentration (equal N) with the following relaxation times is given in the table below as a function of T_R and T_E.

msec	Compartment 1, T_1 = 1600 msec and T_2 = 540 msec; and Compartment 2, T_1 = 600 msec and T_2 = 120 msec					
	Compartment 1			Compartment 2		
	Signal	$1-e^{-T_R/T_1}$	e^{-2T_E/T_2}	Signal	$1-e^{-T_R/T_1}$	e^{-2T_E/T_2}
T_R = 800, T_E = 10	0.38N	0.4	0.96	0.56N	0.7	0.8
T_R = 2000, T_E = 80	0.52N	0.7	0.74	0.29N	0.96	0.3

The conditions T_R = 800, T_E = 10 (sometimes abbreviated in the magnetic resonance literature as 800/10) generate images in which the signal from Compartment 2 (0.56) is larger than that of Compartment 1 (0.38). Compartment 2 will appear brighter in these images, which are heavily T_1 weighted (or attenuated): $1-e^{-T_R/T_1}$ = 0.4 and 0.7. For the 2000/80 image, compartment 1 has the higher signal intensity! This is because of less T_1 attenuation and highly enhanced T_2 weighting:

$$e^{-2T_E/T_2} = 0.7 \text{ and } 0.3.$$

This inversion of the gray scale is common in proton MRI and is due to the combination of the inequality of T_1 and T_2 (intrinsic) and the ability to weight differentially (attenuate) the image intensity through selection of a wide range of values of T_R and T_E.

QUESTIONS FOR SECTIONS 6.4 AND 6.5

Select the one true statement:

1. A spin echo proton image obtained with a long T_R and a short T_E should have a lower signal intensity throughout the image than one obtained with a short T_R and a long T_E.

2. For a constant T_R in spin echo imaging, the image intensity will increase as T_E increases.

3. For a constant T_E in spin echo imaging, the image intensity will either stay the same or decrease with increasing T_R.

4. For a tissue whose various compartments have T_1 values near 900 msec and T_2 values near 300 msec, the spin echo imaging sequence with T_R = 450 msec and T_E = 20 msec can be said to be heavily T_1 weighted (attenuated).

5. For a tissue whose various compartments have T_1 values near 1200 msec and T_2 values near 200 msec, the spin echo imaging sequence with T_R = 1200 msec and T_E = 2 msec can be said to be heavily T_2 weighted (attenuated).

6.6 Lipid or Fat Protons Contribute to the Intensity in Proton Magnetic Resonance Images, But Not Those of the Brain

Thus far in our discussion of proton MRIs we have restricted our attention to water protons. Of course water protons make the major contribution to the intensity of clinical proton images, and the sole contribution to those of the brain. This results from the high abundance of water in tissue, and because the water molecule is small and has a relatively long intrinsic T_2—its FID persists for a relatively long time, thereby generating an intense magnetic resonance signal. Lipids or fats also are highly abundant in tissue, especially in cell membranes. Having fatty acids (Diagram 6-1) as major constituents, lipids should also contribute strongly to the intensity of proton MRIs. In most normal tissue they exhibit extremely short intrinsic T_2 values because they are tightly packed into membrane structures and restricted in the range and mobility of motion. Therefore, this dampens the FID so that only a relatively weak proton signal is usually generated. For example, suppose that water in a tissue sample exhibits an intrinsic T_2 of 150 msec, whereas, under the same conditions, protons in the lipid fatty acids exhibit an intrinsic T_2 of 20 msec. For a spin echo imaging technique with $T_E = 20$ msec, the T_2 (intrinsic) weighting or attenuation factor in the image intensity is $e^{-40/150} = 0.75$ for water protons and $e^{-40/20} = 0.14$ for lipid fatty acid protons. This means that, even if the water and lipid fatty acid T_1's and proton spin densities (N) were equal, the water proton contribution to the image intensity would exceed that of lipid fatty acid protons by more than a factor of 5 ($5 \times 0.14 = 0.70 < 0.75$). In the case of brain tissue, despite the high proton concentration of lipid of white matter, the lipid proton intrinsic T_2 values are so short that they make *no* detectable contribution to the intensity of brain proton images.

Why are the tissue lipid proton intrinsic T_2 values so short? Recall from Chapter 5 that the ability of an agent to dephase proton spins depends on the presence of a *large magnetic moment that persists for a long period of time*. In this respect cell membrane lipids exhibit closely packed magnetized segments that are very effective in the rapid irreversible dephasing of proton spins nearby (Fig. 6-6). In some disease states (e.g., tumors), cell membrane lipids are loosely packed, intrinsic T_2 relaxation is slower, the lipid CH_2 magnetization persists longer, and the CH_2 protons make an enhanced contribution to the image intensity.

$$HO\overset{\overset{\textstyle O}{\|}}{C} - (CH_2)_n - CH_3 \ (N = 16+)$$ DIAGRAM 6-1. Structure of a fatty acid.

FIG. 6-6 *follows next page.*

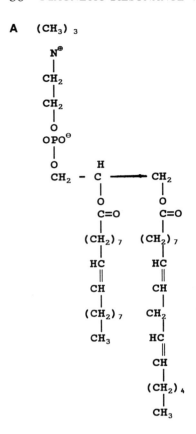
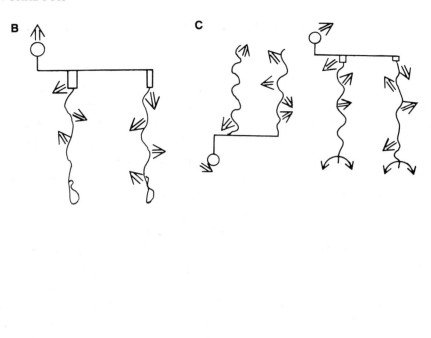

FIG. 6-6. Lipids: structure, segmental magnetization, and dilayer organization. **A:** Structure of a lipid. **B:** Schematic of a lipid structure with magnetized segments induced by the B_0 field. **C:** Schematic of a lipid bilayer of the cell membrane. Segmental motion in the bilayer is highly restricted, magnetic "contacts" persist for a long time, and intrinsic T_2 relaxation is rapid (T_2 is short).

QUESTIONS FOR SECTION 6.6

Select the one true statement:

1. The intensity in spin echo proton images is determined solely by the water content of the tissue imaged.

2. Lipid protons never make contributions to the intensity of proton images of tissue.

3. Lipids organized in membranes usually have a limited range and mobility of motion because they are tightly packed.

4. Lipid protons in tissue generally have longer T_1 and T_2 values than water protons in the same tissue.

5. e^{-1} is a smaller number than e^{-20}.

7

Frequency, Phase, and Image Construction Revisited

It is appropriate to conclude this introductory text on proton magnetic resonance imaging (MRI) by revisiting the concepts of signal frequency and phase for the purpose of showing more explicitly, but still in a qualitative manner, how these two important parameters are used to encode position of the proton density. In this discussion *we will neglect relaxation effects* and will be concerned with only nine picture elements (pixels) in the images considered. A schematic image is illustrated in Fig. 7-1, in which the pixels form a matrix with rows along the y axis and columns along the x axis. To simplify the discussion further, we have assigned the same proton density to pixels in each of the columns as noted in the figure (Column 1 = 1, Column 2 = 0.33, and Column 3 = 0.20). Note that the pixel dimensions (ordinarily ~1 mm × 1 mm) are exaggerated in Fig. 7-1 and the figures that follow so that information can be recorded conveniently. We have projected the pixels onto the xy plane in which the protons are at resonance after a slice selection gradient along the z axis and a frequency selective radiofrequency (RF) pulse have been turned on, and then off. In effect the task in constructing the image is to find out how much proton density is in each of the pixels. We already know but are working the problem backward to illustrate how the image was constructed in the first place.

Proton density can be assigned to each of the columns, 1, 2, and 3, by turning on a linear field gradient along the x axis while the proton signal is collected. An ideal free induction decay (FID) that would constitute the signal during the imposition of a linear field gradient of 0.2 G/cm is re-

87

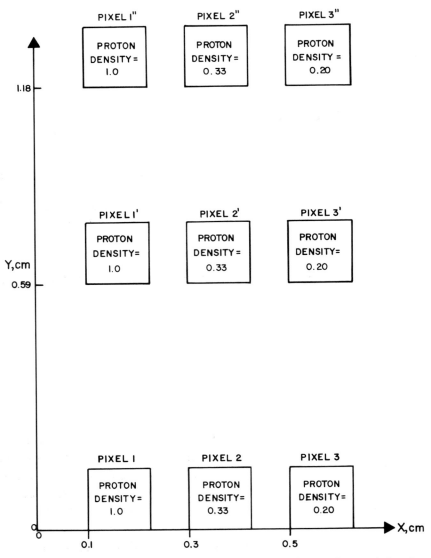

FIG. 7-1. Schematic of a proton image with 9 pixels (picture elements) forming 3 columns along the x axis (frequency-encoding axis) and 3 rows along the y axis (phase-encoding axis). The relative proton densities of Columns 1, 2, and 3 are 1:0.33:0.20. The pixel sizes (~1 mm × 1 mm) are exaggerated in this figure and the ones that follow.

produced in Fig. 7-2A. Only two cycles of the FID are shown—relaxation effects being neglected, the FID continues forever. Our reference point on the x axis is a landmark at 0 cm at which the field is, say, 1.0000000 T, where the precessional frequency is 42.57 MHz. We will define this as 0 frequency and measure the frequency of the protons in Columns 1, 2, and 3 with respect to it. The pixels in Column 1 are 0.1 cm from our reference point on the x axis and, compared to the reference point, the static magnet field is .02 G (.1 cm × 0.2 G/cm) higher. This corresponds to .000002 T and the precessional frequency of the protons in the pixels in Column 1 will be 85.1 Hz $\left(0.000002 \text{ T} \times 42.57 \dfrac{\text{MHz}}{\text{T}}\right)$ *higher* than the reference point. Proceeding in a similar fashion, it can be shown that, compared to the reference point, the protons in pixels in Column 2 will

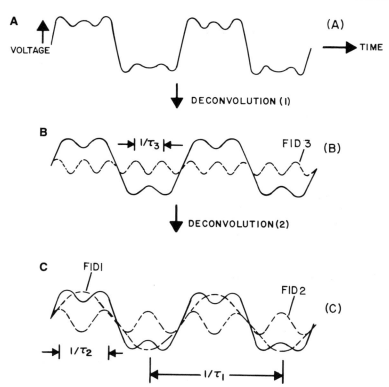

FIG. 7-2. Frequency encoding of the x position of the pixel columns of FIG. 7-1 by turning on a linear field gradient (0.2 G/cm) during acquisition of the FID. **A:** Complex FID composed of three "signals". **B:** Deconvolution of the complex FID into a high-frequency component, FID 3 of pixel column 3, and the composite FID of pixel columns 1 and 2. **C:** Deconvolution into the remaining two components, FID 1 of pixel column 2 and FID 2 of pixel column 2. The relative amplitudes of FID 1, FID 2, and FID 3 are 1:0.33:0.20. The frequency of FID 3 is 423.7 Hz, which is: 1 divided by the time required to complete 1 cycle, or $1/\tau_3$, where $\tau_3 = 2.34$ msec. τ_1 is 11.75 msec with an FID 1 frequency of 85.1 Hz and τ_2 is 3.91 msec with an FID 2 frequency of 255.4 Hz.

experience a higher field of 0.06 G and a higher frequency of 255.4 Hz, and the protons in pixels in Column 3 will experience a higher field of 0.1 G and a higher frequency of 425.7 Hz.

What the detector should see is a composite or convoluted FID, which is the sum of an FID of relative intensity 1 at 85.1 Hz, an FID of relative intensity 0.33 at 255.4 Hz, and an FID of relative intensity 0.20 at 425.7 Hz. Figs. 7-2B and C illustrate the stepwise deconvolution of the complex FID of Fig. 7-2A into three such signals of the appropriate intensities and frequencies. As depicted in Fig. 7-3, this operation provides only a projection of the proton density along the x axis (the frequency-encoding or read-out axis) since all pixels in a given pixel column have the same frequency and phase.

The phase-encoding gradient that is turned on, then off, along the y axis *before* the acquisition of the FID provides the information about the proton density in the rows of pixels along the y axis. For example, consider a y phase-encoding gradient of amplitude 0.05 G/cm applied for 1 msec and then turned off, before acquisition of the FID. The effect of the y gradient

90 MAGNETIC RESONANCE WORKBOOK

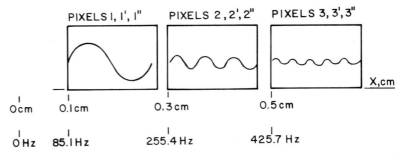

FIG. 7-3. The one-dimensional representation of the schematic image of FIG. 7-1, "created" by turning on a field gradient of 0.2 G/cm during acquisition of the composite FID shown in FIG. 7-2A. The phase-encoding gradient was not turned on before the FID was acquired. Again, note that the pixel sizes have been exaggerated so that the FID can be displayed conveniently in the pixels.

will be to shift the phase of the signals in direct proportion to the y coordinate. For pixels 1″, 2″, and 3″ the y coordinate is 1.18 cm and for a gradient of 0.05 G/cm, these pixels will experience a field that is 0.059 G(.05 G/cm × 1.18 cm) or 0.0000059 T higher than the field at the y reference point, which is also where the 1, 2, and 3 pixels are located. This means that the precessional frequencies of pixels 1″, 2″, and 3″ will be 250 Hz (0.0000059 T × 42.57 MHz/T = 0.00025 MHz = 250 Hz) higher than the precessional frequencies of pixels 1, 2, and 3. If the field gradient is turned on for 1 msec (0.001 sec) and then turned off, pixels 1″, 2″, and 3″ will have gained 0.25 cycles of phase with respect to pixels 1, 2, and 3 $\left(250 \frac{\text{cycles}}{\text{sec}} \times 0.001 \text{ sec} = 0.25 \text{ cycles}\right)$. This is illustrated in Fig. 7-4 where it is also shown that pixels 1′, 2′, and 3′, which are at y coordinate 0.59 cm, only gain 0.125 cycles of phase with respect to pixels 1, 2, and 3 in the field gradient of 0.05 G/cm. Thus, each pixel has acquired a unique frequency and phase through the use of the two appropriately timed gradients of the static magnetic field.

We have worked this example "backward" to provide some insight into how the static field gradients must be used and how the FIDs must be processed to interrogate the proton density and assign it to the appropriate pixels. The *actual* process of image construction is complicated by our inability to examine the proton density in each row of pixels along the y axis separately. When a field gradient is applied along the y axis, each row of pixels acquires a specific phase and all of this phase information across the entire imaging plane is read out (contained) in the acquired FID. For example, the intensity, phase, and frequency data represented in Fig. 7-4 is a snapshot of the individual pixels after the:

–imaging plane has been selected with the appropriate z static field gradient and frequency selective RF pulse turned on, then off
–phase-encoding y gradient, 0.05 G/cm, has been turned on for 1 msec, then turned off
–frequency-encoding (x) gradient has just been turned on.

What the detector sees, however, is not the individual pixels, but the sum

FREQUENCY, PHASE, AND IMAGE CONSTRUCTION 91

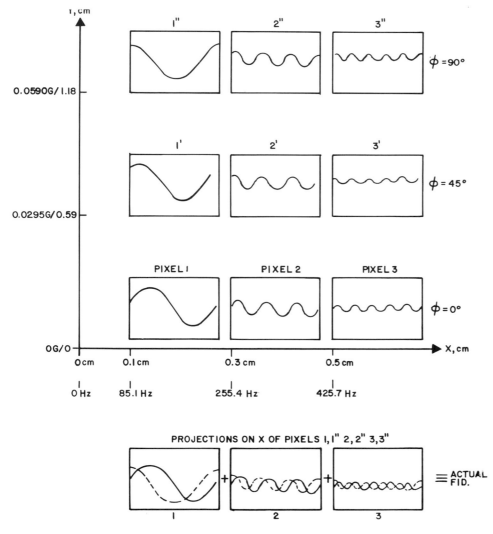

FIG. 7-4. The 2D representation of the schematic image of FIG. 7-1 "created" by turning on a field of 0.05 G/cm along the y axis for 1 msec and then turning it off. A frequency-encoding gradient of 0.2 G/cm was then turned on along the x axis during acquisition of the FID. The y gradient shifted the phase of the pixels 1', 2', and 3' by 45° and the phase of pixels 1", 2", and 3" by 90° with respect to the pixels 1, 2, and 3. Also shown are the projections 1, 2, and 3 on the x axis. These projections are the sum of pixels 1 and 1", 2 and 2", and 3 and 3", respectively. For the sake of clarity in the drawings, the contribution of pixels 1', 2', and 3' to the projections have been omitted.

of the information in each of the columns projected onto the x (frequency-encoding, or read-out) axis presented as an FID which is a composite or sum of the FIDs in each of the individual columns 1, 2, and 3. The projections of the FIDs of pixels 1, 1", 2, 2", and 3, 3" onto the x axis are shown in Fig. 7-4 (the projections of the 1', 2', and 3' have not been included to avoid cluttering the drawing). The actual FID will be a sum of projections 1, 2, and 3.

In *constructing an image* with the aid of a powerful computer, the processes we employ are, in a way, just the reverse of the steps we have been considering. The actual FID of Fig. 7-4 is deconvoluted into a set of frequency components (projections) on the frequency-encoding (x) axis in a manner similar to that illustrated in Fig. 7-2. The next step would be to deconvolute the phase data in the FIDs in each of the columns 1, 2, and 3 into a specific intensity for each of the rows. However, there is not sufficient information to do this with the data obtained from the application of only one phase-encoding gradient. Additional phase-encoding information such as that depicted in Fig. 7-5 must be obtained. As shown in the figure, a field gradient of amplitude 0.1 G/cm applied for 1 msec before the application of the read-out gradient would shift the phase of pixels 1″, 2″, and 3″ by 180° and that of the pixels 1′, 2′, and 3′ by 90°. This would result in a much different set of frequency deconvoluted FIDs projected

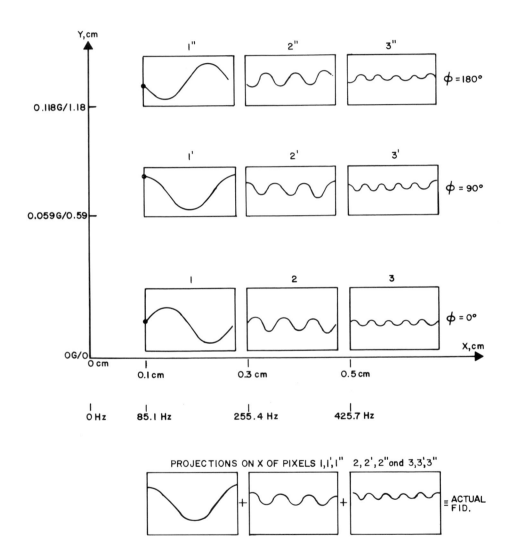

FIG. 7-5. The 2D representation of the schematic image of FIG. 7-1 "created" by turning on a field gradient of 0.1 G/cm along the y axis for 1 msec and then turning it off. Then a frequency-encoding gradient of 0.2 G/cm was turned on along the x axis during acquisition of the FID. When the y gradient (the phase-encoding gradient) was turned on, pixels 1′, 2′, and 3′ gained 90° of phase (Φ) and pixels 1″, 2″, and 3″ gained 180° of phase with respect to pixels 1, 2, and 3. The projections on the frequency-encoding x axis are deceptively simple frequency deconvoluted FIDs because pixels 1 and 1″, 2 and 2″, and 3 and 3″ are 180° out of phase with a resultant concellation of signal intensities from these rows.

onto the x axis in the columns 1, 2, and 3, as shown in Fig. 7-5. If we now compared in detail the projections in Fig. 7-2 (0 field gradient), Fig. 7-4 (0.05 G/cm field gradient), and Fig. 7-5, we could reconstruct the image of Fig. 7-1 where the proton density is assigned to the appropriate pixels because each pixel is characterized by a unique frequency and phase.

In the more general case of image construction, 128, 256, or 512 frequency-encoding elements (columns) are used to obtain high resolution on the x axis. As noted before, we would need as many phase-encoding steps to produce equivalent resolution on the y axis. The necessary phase data would be acquired by stepping the amplitude of the phase-encoding gradient through 128, 256, or 512 increments and after each increment: acquiring the FID with the frequency-encoding gradient on; deconvoluting the FID with respect to the frequency projections; and storing the frequency deconvoluted phase and intensity information in the appropriate projection column in a computer. The computer could then deconvolute the phase and intensity information for each column (1, 2, 3 . . . n) into the appropriate rows in a manner similar to that illustrated in Fig. 7-2, where instead of frequency, phase is the dependent variable. The two-dimensional (2D) deconvolution described here qualitatively is commonly referred to as a 2D Fourier transformation (FT). We will be considering FT methods in more detail in subsequent elementary textbooks.

In conclusion, we note briefly some complications in the simple models we have developed. These will be treated in appropriate detail in future texts in this series. First, the pixels have a finite width, usually 1 mm $\times$ 1 mm. Consequently they will be characterized by a narrow band of frequencies and phases rather than by a single frequency and phase. For example, the pixels in Fig. 7-3 will have a frequency width of 85.1 Hz (0.00002 T/cm $\times$ 0.1 cm $\times$ 42.57 10^{+6} Hz/T = 85.1 Hz). The finite band widths do not present especially difficult problems in receiver design or in computer analysis of the data.

Second, the timing diagram in Fig. 6-5 is oversimplified in the characterization of the shape of the slice selection gradient G_z as ⊓. This neglects the facts that the width of the slice is finite and the frequency selective pulse persists for a relatively long time, about 1 msec or longer. These realities lead to a dephasing of magnetization across the slice during its selection. For example, the two sides of a 5-mm slice selected in a gradient of 1 G/cm will differ in precessional frequency by 2129 Hz (0.0001 T/cm $\times$ 0.5 cm $\times$ 42.57 10^{+6} Hz/T = 2129 Hz). If a frequency selective pulse that excites the slice magnetization is left on for 1 msec, then the magnetization on the two sides of the slice will differ in phase by 2.129 cycles (2129 cycles/sec $\times$ 10^{-3} sec = 2.129 cycles). However, this magnetization can be rephased if the static field gradient is reversed for a short time immediately after cessation of the slice selective pulse—in the reversed gradient, the formerly high frequency side of the slice becomes the low frequency side and vice versa. This gradient reversal is denoted in the literature with the symbol ⊓⊔ .

Finally, in this treatment we have completely neglected the oscillating electric fields that necessarily accompany the RF magnetic fields. Electric field effects are particularly important in the design of RF coils and in the consideration of the RF power absorption by biological specimens.

PROBLEMS FOR CHAPTER 7

In working through the problems for Chapter 7 we will need to work with Figs. 7-6 and 7-7.

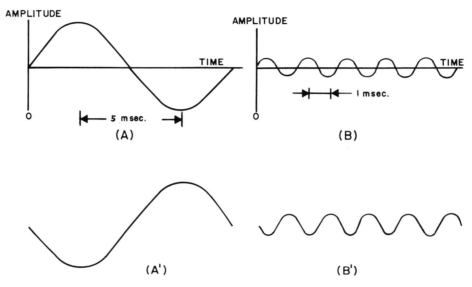

FIG. 7-6. FIDs for working problems 1 through 4.

1. Calculate the frequencies of the proton resonances, relative to the landmark reference assigned as 0 Hz, which give the FIDs reproduced in pixels (A) and (B) of Fig. 7-6.

2. The FIDs of Figs. 7-6A and B resulted from the deconvolution of a composite FID of tissue obtained during the imposition of a frequency-encoding gradient of 0.1 G/cm. What is the distance of the point in the tissue corresponding to pixel A from the reference point that is assigned the frequency 0 Hz? What is the distance between tissue structures corresponding to pixel A and pixel B? Recall that the magnetogyric ratio of the proton is 42.57 $\frac{MHz}{T}$ and that to work the problem, it is probably best to convert the frequency-encoding gradient to Hz/cm.

3. What is the proton density of pixel (A) relative to pixel (B) in Fig. 7-6?

4. In Fig. 7-6 pixel A' is in the same frequency-encoding column as A, and pixel B' is in the same frequency-encoding column as B. A' and B' are in the same phase-encoding row of the image matrix along the y axis and represent coordinates in the tissue that are 1 cm from the AB row. How long would a phase-encoding gradient of 0.1 G/cm need to be applied to cause the observed phase changes between pixel A and A' and pixel B and B'?

Continued on facing page.

PROBLEMS FOR CHAPTER 7 *continued*

5. In Fig. 7-7 there is a schematic column of eight pixels at a specific frequency-encoding location along the x axis. The phase shifts that occur from pixel n to pixel n + 7 were generated by the imposition of a linear phase-encoding gradient along the y axis. Something is wrong with one of the pixels. What is it? Sketch what should be in that pixel. Where should the incorrect pixel be located?

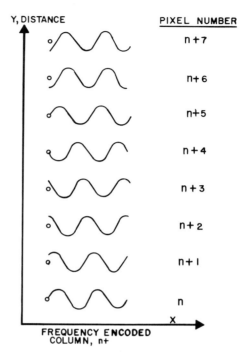

FIG. 7-7. FIDs in the column of eight pixels for working problem 5.

8

The Effect of the Repetition Time T_R and The Echo Evolution Time T_E on Contrast in Simple Spin Echo Proton Images of the Head

In this chapter we provide examples of the effect of the pulse timing parameters T_R and T_E on contrast and signal intensity in simple spin echo images of the head. The timing diagram of the pulse sequences used is sketched in Fig. 6-5. For purposes of the qualitative examination of the images in this section, the following table, which provides *approximate* values of relaxation times and maximum proton densities observable in a spin echo image, is useful. The images in Figs. 8-1 through 8-3 illustrate the extremes of contrast attainable in practice with heavy T_2 and T_1 attenuation (weighting). Recall that the relative contribution of a given tissue to the intensity I of a spin echo image is a product of the proton density N(H) and the T_1 and T_2 attenuation (weighting) factors:

$$I = \text{proton density } (T_1 \text{ attenuation factor}) (T_2 \text{ attenuation factor})$$

$$I = N(H)(1 - e^{-T_R/T_1})e^{-2T_E/T_2}.$$

The heavy T_2 weighting achieved with $T_R = 3000$ msec and $2T_E = 160$ msec (Fig. 8-1) assures that only cerebrospinal fluid (CSF) makes a major contribution to the image intensity (T_2 attenuation factor $= e^{-160/300} = e^{-0.52} = 0.6$) because the T_2 attenuation factors for the other brain con-

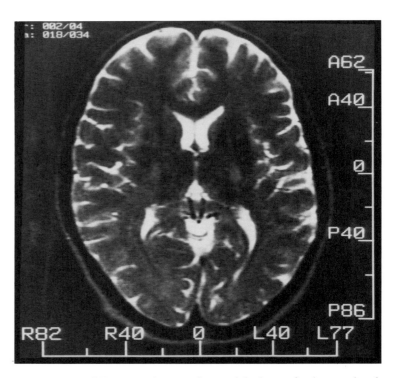

FIG. 8-1. 1.5-T proton image of an axial plane of a human head. The image obtained on a General Electric Medical Systems Signa unit is heavily T_2 weighted: $T_R = 3000$ msec and $2T_E = 160$ msec.

stituents are so small, e.g., white matter 0.1 ($e^{-160/70}$) and gray matter 0.17 ($e^{-160/90}$). In addition, scalp makes little contribution to the heavily T_2 weighted image ($e^{-160/100} = 0.2$). In contrast, scalp makes a large contribution to the heavily T_1 attenuated image (Fig. 8-2) because its T_1 attenuation factor is larger [$(1 - e^{-600/170}) = 0.97$] than those of CSF [$(1 - e^{-600/2000}) = 0.25$], gray matter [$(1 - e^{-600/900}) = 0.5$] or white matter [$(1 - e^{-600/600}) = 0.67$]. Because of the way the image intensity is scaled, CSF actually appears black in the heavily T_1 weighted image. In the image with small T_1 attenuation and moderate T_2 attenuation (Fig. 8-3), all components make appreciable contributions to the image intensity with a consequent further altering of the contrast among the components.

The T_1 and T_2 values listed in Table 1 should not be taken literally. Although the relaxation times measured by a given investigator on a given imaging system do show a pronounced tissue dependence that reflect tissue-specific contributions to water relaxation rates, the unfortunate reality at the present stage of development of proton magnetic resonance imaging (MRI) is that different investigators using different imaging systems frequently report markedly different absolute values of T_1 and T_2 for a given tissue. This could reflect instrument specific systematic errors; volume averaging effects; and use of different pulse sequences, regions of interest, and controls who were not age matched. An additional complication is that, unlike normal brain, most tissues contain both water and fat proton contributions to the MRI signal. These protons have markedly different T_1 and T_2 values, but usually only the average is observed, an average

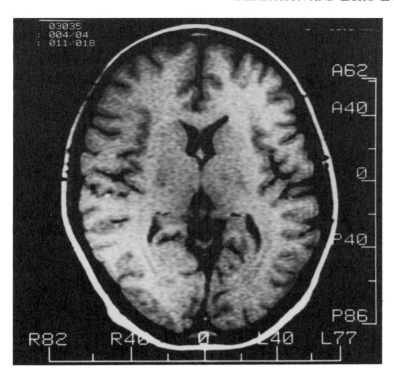

FIG. 8-2. 1.5-T proton image of the same axial plane as in FIG. 8-1, but this image is heavily T_1 weighted: $T_R = 600$ and $2T_E = 20$ msec.

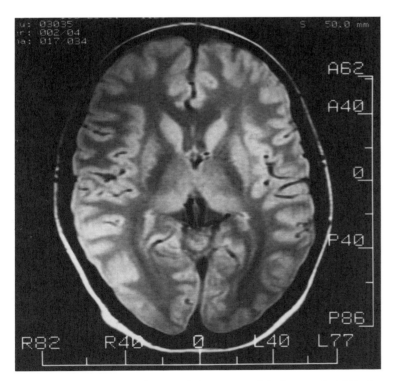

FIG. 8-3. 1.5-T proton image of the same axial plane as in FIG. 8-1, but this image is only moderately weighted by relaxation times: $T_R = 3000$ and $2T_E = 20$ msec. This resembles the actual distribution of proton spin density.

TABLE 1. *APPROXIMATE RELAXATION TIMES AND MAXIMUM OBSERVABLE PROTON DENSITIES OF TISSUE IN VIVO AT A STATIC MAGNETIC FIELD OF 1.5 T*

"Tissue"	Maximum Observable Proton Density (Relative)	Approximate T_1 (msec)	Relaxation Times T_2 (msec)
CSF	1.0	2000.	300.
Gray Matter	0.9	900.	90.
White Matter	0.8	600.	70.
"Scalp"	0.7	170.	100.

that depends on the water and fat composition of the tissue. Nonetheless, the approximate relaxation times are a useful guide to the origin of the variations in intensity in proton images.

Shown in Fig. 8-4 are images that illustrate further the effect on the appearance of proton images of pulse timing parameters and the selection of the gray scale range and brightness levels for preparing hard copies. Again, the T_2 weighted images (Figs. 8-4A,B) have large contributions from

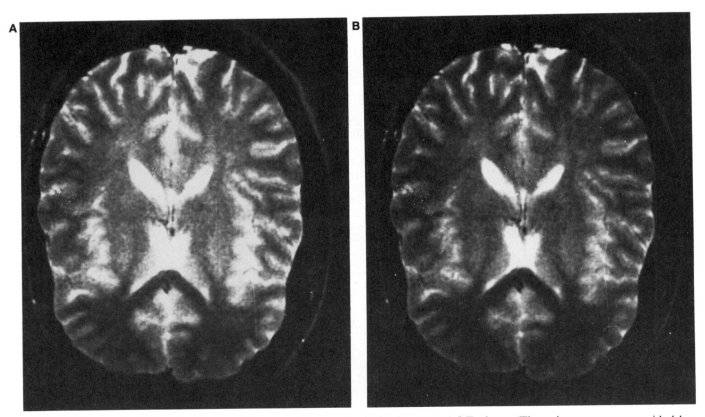

FIG. 8-4. A set of axial proton images of a normal human brain in the same 1.5-T plane. (These images were provided by R.R. Sibbitt, M.D., Director, Sante Fe Imaging Center, Santa Fe, New Mexico, and were obtained on the Siemens Magnetom.) The pulse timing parameters (msec) are: **A, B,** $T_R = 2500$ and $2T_E = 90$; **C, D,** $T_R = 450$ and $2T_E = 22$; **E, F,** $T_R = 2500$ and $2T_E = 22$. For each pair of images (**A** and **B** or **C** and **D** or **E** and **F**) the digital pixel information is the same, but the display parameter (gray scale range and brightness levels) have been altered to change the apparent contrast between the image pairs.

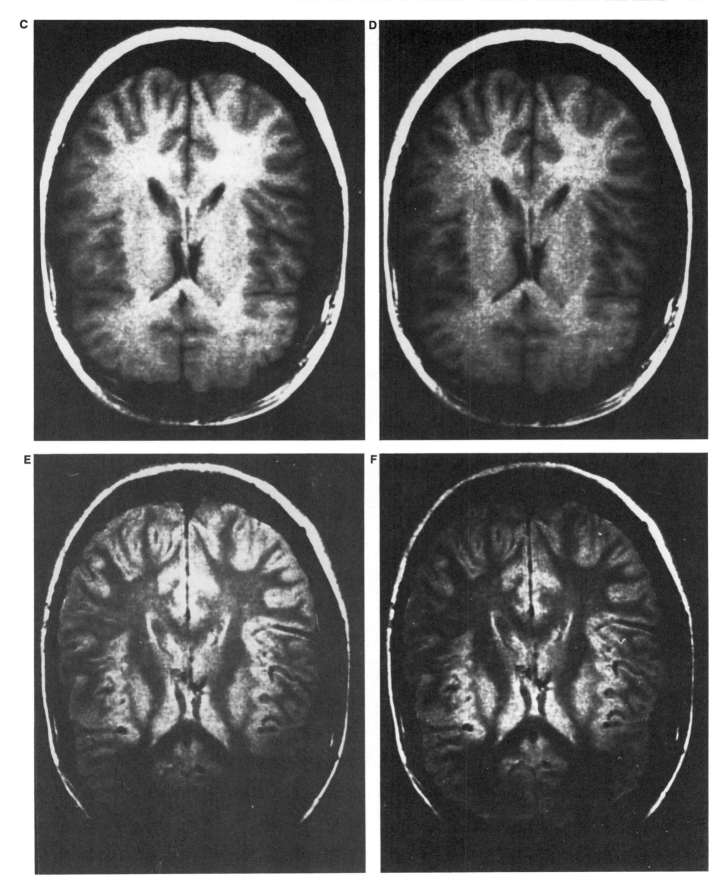

102 MAGNETIC RESONANCE WORKBOOK

CSF and minor contributions from scalp. Although these two images were prepared from the same digital data, the apparent contrast in them is different because the gray scale range (window setting) and brightness level were different. The window sets the intensity range of the image pixel values, whereas the level sets the brightness at which the pixel intensities will be displayed. For example, with too narrow a window setting, all pixel intensities above the upper level of the window setting will appear at the maximum brightness, whereas those below the minimum setting will appear at the minimum intensity (background). Variation of the narrowness of the window setting is used to optimize contrast among various structures in an image.

In the heavily T_1 weighted images (Figs. 8-4C,D), the appearance of dark CSF and bright scalp is again characteristic for proton images of the head. The moderately T_2 weighted images shown in Figs. 8-4E and F closely resemble the actual distribution of proton *density*, where again the apparent contrast is different in the two images because different window settings and brightness levels were used. Note the change in the relative

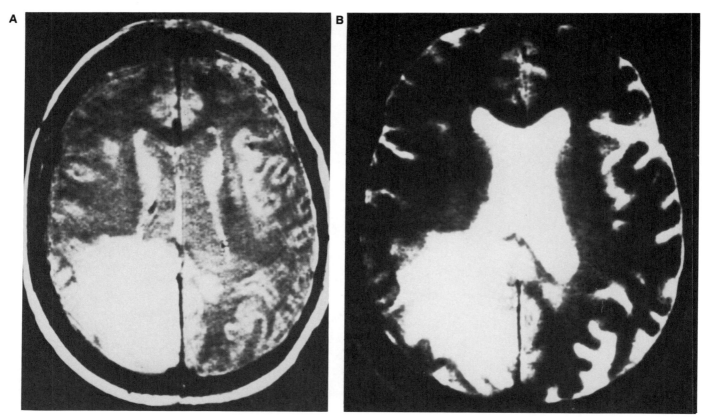

FIG. 8-5. 1.5-T axial proton image of the head of a patient with a glioblastoma of the right occipital lobe postradiation therapy. **A,** "proton density" image $T_R = 2500$ and $2T_E = 22$ msec; **B,** heavily T_2 weighted image, $T_R = 2500$ and $2T_E = 90$ msec; **C,** heavily T_1 weighted image, $T_R = 450$ and $T_E = 22$ msec. (These images were provided by R.R. Sibbitt, M.D., Director, Santa Fe Imaging Center, Santa Fe, New Mexico.)

intensities of gray and white matter in the heavily T_1 weighted images (Figs. 8-4C,D) and the proton density images (Figs. 8-4E,F). Because gray matter has a longer T_1 value than white matter, its intensity is more highly attenuated in the T_1 weighted image.

Fig. 8-5 contains a set of proton images of the same axial plane of a patient presenting after radiation therapy of a glioblastoma of the right occipital lobe. The area of the tumor and associated edema is evident from its brightness on the spin density (Fig. 8-4A) and the heavily T_2 weighted (Fig. 8-5B) image and its darkness on the heavily T_1 weighted image (Fig. 8-5C). It is apparent from these intensity changes that the tumor water T_1 and T_2 values are much larger than those for water in normal brain tissue. Note that, especially in the heavily T_1 weighted image, there is an alternating pattern of hypointense and hyperintense rings. These "ghosts" in the head images of this patient, who was not able to remain motionless, are artifacts resulting from a reinforcement and cancellation of phase-encoded signals misregistered because of the motion (see also problem 7.4).

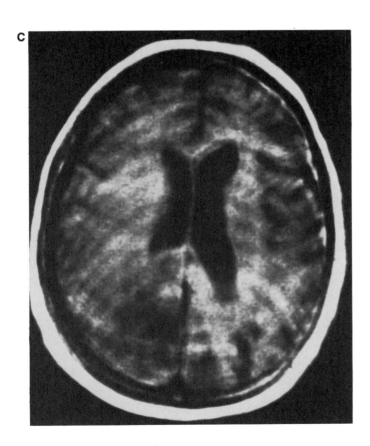

Question for Chapter 8 next page

QUESTION FOR CHAPTER 8

The proton image shown in Fig. 8-6 was obtained from the same patient whose proton images were shown in Fig. 8-5. The image was obtained after the intravenous injection of an aqueous solution of a paramagnetic contrast agent (~0.1 mmole/1 kg), which changes the relaxation times of water in the tissue in which it transiently accumulates. In the brain, this contrast agent, aqueous Gadolinium diethylenetriaminepentaacetic acid (GdDTPA) transiently accumulates in regions of disruption of the blood brain barrier, regions that are obvious from a comparison of Figs. 8-5 and 8-6. Why does this comparison suggest that GdDTPA dramatically lowers the T_1 of water?

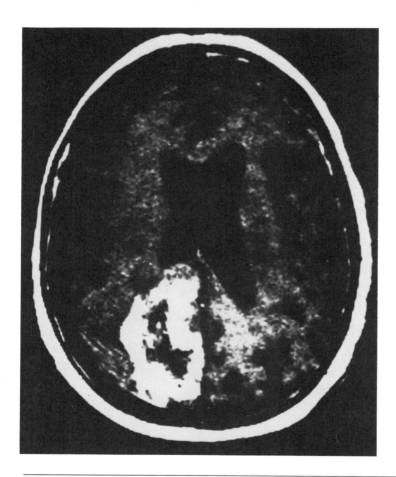

FIG. 8-6. 1.5-T proton image for the patient of FIG. 8-5 after administration of a paramagnetic contrast agent, GdDTPA.

9
Review Questions

Set A

The following table of values of e^{-x} will be helpful in answering the questions in Set A.

x	e^{-x}
0	1.000
0.1	0.905
0.2	0.819
0.5	0.607
0.6	0.549
0.7	0.500
1.0	0.368
2.0	0.135
3.0	0.050
4.0	0.02

1. A tissue has a T_1 of 900 msec and a T_2 of 90 msec. The tissue is proton imaged using one pulse sequence with a $T_R = 900$ msec and a $T_E = 45$ msec (900/45), and then imaged with an 1800/90 pulse sequence.

a. Which pulse sequence should result in a higher proton intensity in the image?
b. Which image is more heavily T_1 attenuated?
c. Which image is more heavily T_2 attenuated?
d. Which image requires more time to obtain?
e. If 256 phase-encoding steps are used for both images, how long would it take to obtain the data for the 1800/90 and 900/45 pulse sequences?

2. At a static field strength $B_0 = 0.35$ T, liver has a $T_1 = 450$ msec and $T_2 = 50$ msec, whereas adipose tissue has $T_1 = 225$ msec and $T_2 = 50$ msec. Which of the following pulse sequences will produce images with the higher intensity ratio between liver and adjacent fat: (a) 450/25 or (b) 900/25 (assume that the proton density in liver and fat is the same)? Which

of the two sequences would you use if a distinction between adipose tissue and liver were important in the examination?

3. At a static field strength $B_0 = 0.35$ T, spleen has $T_1 = 900$ msec and $T_2 = 100$ msec and adjacent tissue has $T_1 = 225$ msec and $T_2 = 50$ msec. Which of the following pulse sequences will produce images with the higher intensity ratio between spleen and adjacent tissue: (a) 900/100 or (b) 900/50? Which pulse sequence would be preferred in routine diagnostic imaging?

4. One tissue compartment (1) has $T_1 = 1000$ msec and $T_2 = 100$ msec. An adjacent tissue compartment (2) with the same proton density has $T_1 = 500$ msec and $T_2 = 50$ msec. Verify that (a) the pulse sequence 5000/50 results in proton images with a larger intensity ratio between the adjacent tissues than (b) a pulse sequence 1000/50. Nonetheless, if these were the only imaging sequences available, why would the 1000/50 sequence be the one of choice for routine diagnostic imaging?

5. Consider again the tissues of Problem 4 above. The pulse sequence 1000/200 produces proton images with a much larger intensity ratio between adjacent compartments than the sequences 1000/50. Nonetheless, if these were the only pulse sequences available, why would the sequence of choice for routine diagnostic imaging be 1000/50?

Set B

Mark the statement true or false.

1. Magnets slowly induce a permanent magnetization in body tissue.

2. The strength of a static magnetic field (B_0) is measured in units of Gauss or Tesla.

3. If the resonance frequency of the proton dipole is 42.57 MHz in a 1.0 T B_0 field, then its resonance frequency in a 2.0 T B_0 field will be 21.28 MHz.

4. If an alternating current (AC) is passed through a radiofrequency (RF) coil, an oscillating magnetic field is created perpendicular to the AC.

5. A RF coil cannot be used both to excite tissue protons to resonance and to detect the tissue proton resonance signal.

6. A head coil is larger than a body RF coil.

7. The precession of a magnetic dipole inside a sensitive RF coil can create a direct current in the coil.

8. A free induction decay (FID) consisting of a sine wave that repeats itself every second has a higher frequency than one that repeats itself every millisecond.

9. One cycle/second is 1 MHz.

10. One cycle/second is equivalent to 2π radians/second.

11. The frequency of a proton magnetic resonance signal can be changed by changing the strength of the magnetic field experienced by the protons already at resonance in an imaging plane.

12. The phase and frequency of a proton magnetic resonance signal cannot be changed after the protons in an imaging plane selected have been excited to resonance.

13. Both the phase and frequency of a proton magnetic resonance signal can be determined in a proton imaging study.

14. A selective RF pulse contains only a narrow range of frequencies.

15. The phase of a proton magnetic resonance signal with a $0°$ phase shift is the same as that having a $360°$ phase shift.

16. One cycle contains $180°$.

17. A π pulse is a $90°$ pulse.

18. With present-day technology, higher strength magnetic fields can be achieved with superconducting coils than with materials having a permanent magnetism.

19. The larger the strength of a static magnetic field is, the larger are the associated fringe fields that can affect certain types of pacemakers and television screens, and which can accelerate ferromagnetic objects like screwdrivers and scalpels into the center of the magnet.

20. The shape and size of RF coils have little effect on the appearance of proton magnetic resonance images (MRIs).

21. Magnets for MRI systems must be reasonably homogeneous, a state that usually can be attained by a combination of passive and active shimming.

22. For the same tissue sample, the more homogeneous the static magnetic field is the longer the proton FID persists.

23. The more effective the intrinsic spin-spin relaxation of a tissue is (the shorter the intrinsic spin-spin relaxation time is), the shorter is the period of time that the proton FID persists.

24. Spin-lattice relaxation (T_1) processes not only lead to recovery of z magnetization but they also serve to remove magnetization from the xy plane.

25. In aqueous solutions, proteins and water molecules have a wide range of rates of rotation and collision.

26. Magnetic fields intrinsic to tissue and fluctuating at the Larmor frequency are not effective in promoting spin-lattice relaxation.

Set B *continued*

27. Spin-lattice relaxation of water protons in aqueous solutions involves a transfer of energy from proton magnetic dipoles to the water "lattice".

28. Spin-lattice relaxation of water proton dipoles usually occurs at a faster rate in aqueous protein solutions than in pure water itself.

29. Proteins in aqueous solutions are not effective in accelerating spin-lattice relaxation of water protons.

30. Spin-lattice relaxation is an exponential process in which the initial stages of recovery of magnetization along the z axis occur more slowly than the final stages of recovery.

31. The time constant for spin-spin relaxation is called T_2 and it is the time when magnetization in the xy plane has decayed to approximately $\frac{1}{3}$ its initial value.

32. In tissue samples, the T_2 of water protons is always equal to or less than T_1.

33. In general it is true that the greater the resolution required in the phase-encoding direction, the more time required to obtain a proton image.

34. In general it is true that the greater the resolution required in the frequency-encoding direction, the more time required to obtain a proton image.

35. In proton MRI, the selection of T_R to be much greater than T_1 ensures that the z magnetization will fully recover between phase-encoding steps.

36. A protein in aqueous solution exhibits slower motion than water molecules.

37. Dephasing of water proton dipoles at resonance by fluctuating internal magnetic fields caused by dissolved proteins is a random process.

38. Water proton dipoles at resonance, dephased by a random process, can be rephased by a π RF pulse.

39. If a linear phase-encoding gradient of 0.1 G/cm applied for 1 msec causes a phase change of 90° between the FIDs of pixels A and B in the same column along the phase-encoding axis, then a linear phase-encoding gradient of 0.2 G/cm applied for 1 msec will cause a 180° phase shift between the FIDs of the same pixels.

40. For a B_1 field of the same strength, the field must be turned on longer for a 90° pulse than for a 180° pulse.

41. For a sample net magnetization initially aligned along the z (B_0) axis, a B_1 45° pulse generates more magnetization in the xy plane than does a 90° pulse.

42. The pulse sequence, $\pi/2$, wait, π, wait, acquire FID, will result in the same proton magnetic resonance signal as the sequence, π, wait, $\pi/2$, acquire FID.

43. A tissue sample with a long intrinsic T_2 value will have a more persistent (longer lasting) FID than a tissue sample with a short intrinsic T_2 value.

44. The sum of two FIDs, which are identical in amplitude and frequency components, but which are $180°$ out of phase, is zero.

45. If a lesion in a tissue has the same proton density, T_2, and T_1 values as the tissue, then the lesion should exhibit the same intensity as the tissue in proton MRIs no matter what values of T_R and T_E are selected.

46. If a lesion in a tissue has the same proton density and T_2 value as those of the tissue but exhibits a different T_1 value, then the lesion is best distinguished from the tissue using a spin-lattice relaxation attenuated pulsing sequence.

47. If a lesion in a tissue has the same proton density and T_1 values as the tissue but exhibits a different T_2 value, then the lesion is best distinguished from the tissue using a spin-spin relaxation attenuated pulsing sequence.

48. The longer the period of time that two proton magnetic dipoles are in close contact, the more quickly they lose phase coherence owing to magnetic dipolar interactions.

49. The process described in question 48 is a nonrandom process that can be rephased by a π pulse.

50. In the pulse sequence $\pi/2$, T_E, π, T_E, acquire FID, T_R, repeat, T_1 weighting (attenuation) is achieved by shortening T_R (keeping T_E short), and T_2 weighting (attenuation) is achieved by lengthening T_E (keeping T_R long).

Answer Key

CHAPTER 1

1. obtained using invasive techniques
2. gyroscopes
3. slowly induce a permanent magnetization in body tissue
4. has no effect on the appearance of a proton magnetic resonance image
5. is of little utility in proton MRI
6. is a phenomenon unique to proton nuclear dipoles
7. cannot provide information about the spatial location of the proton density

CHAPTER 2

1. has a phase that cannot be shifted or altered
2. moving the patient in the bore of the magnet so that the RF coil can excite a specific slice of protons
3. is the same as that for the signal of a proton that has experienced a 180° phase shift owing to the imposition of a field gradient
4. can be changed by the RF oscillator
5. cannot be changed after the protons in the imaging slice selected have been excited to resonance

CHAPTER 3

1. a microcomputer for processing large data sets
2. must be constructed with superconducting wires

3. is best done at the factory, especially if the imaging site contains large masses of iron near the 5 G line of the magnet
4. human nerves

CHAPTER 4

4.3
1. z, B_0, perpendicular, B_0.
2. static
3. 360°, alternating
4. random

4.4
1. oscillating
2. rotating

4.5
1. same
2. continues to precess about the B_0 field
3. rotation of M about B_0 after B_1 has been turned off

4.6
1. 2π
2. slower
3. $\pi/2$
4. larger
5. larger
6. shorter
7. smaller

4.7
1. less
2. the component of M in the xy plane

112 MAGNETIC RESONANCE WORKBOOK

CHAPTER 5

5.1
1. destroy, restore
2. there is a need to generate sufficient data to ensure the appropriate resolution in phase-encoding direction
3. requires that magnetization preexist or be regenerated along the Z axis

5.2
3

5.3
2

5.4
4

5.5
3,6

5.6
2,3

CHAPTER 6

6.1
3,4

6.2
3,4

6.3
2

6.4, 6.5
4

6.6
3

CHAPTER 7

7.1
Pixel A:

$$\text{frequency} = \frac{0.5 \text{ cycles}}{0.005 \text{ sec}}$$

$$= 100 \, \frac{\text{cycles}}{\text{sec}} = 100 \text{ Hz}$$

Pixel B:

$$\text{frequency} = \frac{0.5 \text{ cycles}}{0.001 \text{ sec}} = 500 \text{ Hz}$$

7.2
a. Conversion of gradient to Hz/cm for protons

$$0.1 \, \frac{\text{G}}{\text{cm}} \times 0.0001 \, \frac{\text{T}}{\text{G}} \times 42.57 \, \frac{\text{MHz}}{\text{T}}$$

$$= 425.7 \, \frac{\text{Hz}}{\text{cm}}$$

b. The frequency separation of the reference point and the tissue point corresponding to pixel A is 100 Hz. The distance is:

$$100 \text{ Hz} \times \frac{1 \text{ cm}}{425.7 \text{ Hz}} = 0.23 \text{ cm}$$

c. The distance between structures corresponding to pixels A and B is:

$$(\text{frequency pixel B}$$

$$- \text{ frequency pixel A})$$

$$\times \frac{1 \text{ cm}}{425.7 \text{ Hz}} \text{ or } (500 - 100) \times \frac{1}{425.7}$$

$$= 0.94 \text{ cm}$$

7.3
The proton density of pixel A relative to that of pixel B is the ratio of the amplitudes of the FIDs, approximately 5:1.

7.4
The phase shift between pixels A′ and A and between pixels B′ and B is 180°, or 0.5 cycles. A phase-encoding gradient of 0.1 G/cm corresponds to $0.00001 \, \frac{\text{T}}{\text{cm}}$, and since the proton γ is $42.57 \, \frac{\text{MHz}}{\text{T}}$, this corresponds, in turn, to:

$$.0001 \, \frac{\text{T}}{\text{cm}} \times 42.57 \, \frac{\text{MHz}}{\text{T}} = 425.7 \, \frac{\text{Hz}}{\text{cm}}$$

Since the row AB is 1 cm from row A′B′ in the tissue, the precessional frequencies of pixels in row A′B′ will be higher than that of row AB in the 0.1 G/cm gradient by:

$$425.7 \, \frac{\text{Hz}}{\text{cm}} \times 1 \text{ cm}$$

$$= 425.7 \text{ Hz or } 425.7 \, \frac{\text{cycles}}{\text{sec}}$$

If the gradient is turned on for 1 sec, then the proton density in pixels A′B′ will have gained 435.7 cycles of phase with respect to protons in pixels AB. For the former to gain only 0.5 cycles of phase will require that the gradient be turned on for only

$$0.5 \text{ cycles} \times \frac{1 \text{ sec}}{425.7 \text{ cycles}}$$

$$= 0.0012 \text{ sec or } 1.2 \text{ msec}$$

7.5

The change of phase by 45° increments of pixels n through n + 7 is regular and linear with distance along y except for pixel n + 5. Pixel n + 5 has the same phase as pixel n, and by extrapolation pixel n + 8. The phase of pixel n + 5 and the shape of its FID should be intermediate between pixel n + 4 (phase relative to n of 180°) and pixel n + 6 (phase relative to n of 270°).

CHAPTER 8

The image obtained after the administration of the contrast agent (Fig. 8-6) is heavily T_1 attenuated because scalp is bright and CSF is black. However, parts of the lesion appear bright in Fig. 8-6, whereas in the heavily T_1 attenuated image obtained without GdDTPA, those parts of the lesion are dark. Therefore, the contrast agent must have reduced the T_1 of water protons in those parts of the lesion where it accumulated transiently.

CHAPTER 9 (REVIEW QUESTIONS)

Set A

1. The pulse sequence for which T_R and T_E are used is obviously spin echo sequence in which image intensity (I) is given by:

$$I = N(1 - e^{-T_R/T_1})e^{-2T_E/T_2}, \text{ where}$$

N = proton density.

(a) The sequence 900/45 has an image intensity:

$$I = N(1 - e^{-900/900})e^{-90/90}$$

$$= N(1 - 0.368)0.368$$

$$= N(0.632)0.368 = 0.233 \text{ N}.$$

The sequence 1800/90 has an intensity:

$$I = N(1 - e^{-1800/900})e^{-180/90}$$

$$= N(1 - 0.135)0.135$$

$$= N(0.865)0.135 = 0.117 \text{ N}.$$

Therefore the sequence 900/45 will have a higher proton intensity in the image (0.233 > 0.117).

(b) The factor $(1 - e^{-T_R/T_1})$ is the T_1 attenuation (or weighting) factor; the smaller this factor is, the more heavily T_1 attenuated is the image. Therefore the sequence 900/45 is more heavily T_1 attenuated (0.632 < 0.865).

(c) The factor $^{-2T_E/T_2}$ is the T_2 attenuation factor; the smaller this factor is, the more heavily T_2 attenuated is the image. Therefore, the sequence 1800/90 is more heavily T_2 attenuated (0.135 < 0.368).

(d) The image with the 1800/90 pulse sequence T_R is twice that for the 900/45 sequence.

(e) For the 1800/90 sequence, it would take 1.800 sec $\times$ 256 = 461 sec and for the 900/45 sequence 230 sec. Note that within these imaging times, multiimaging planes can be excited sequentially and the data from them collected sequentially. We shall take this subject up in the next textbook.

2. (a) 450/25 intensities:

Liver:

$$I = N(1 - e^{-450/450})e^{-50/50}$$

$$= N(1 - 0.368)(0.368) = 0.23 \text{ N}$$

Adipose tissue:

$$I = N(1 - e^{-450/225})e^{-50/50}$$

$$= N(1 - 0.135)(0.368) = 0.32 \text{ N}$$

Ratio: 0.32/0.23 = 1.39.

(b) 900/25 intensities:

Liver:

$$I = N(1 - e^{-900/450})e^{-50/50}$$

$$= N(1 - 0.135)0.368 = 0.32 \text{ N}$$

Adipose Tissue:

$$I = N(1 - e^{-900/225})e^{-50/50}$$

$$= N(1 - 0.02)0.368 = 0.36 \text{ N}$$

Ratio: 0.36/0.32 = 1.13.

The sequence of choice would be 450/25 because the contrast between liver and fat is higher. An additional benefit is that the imaging time is shorter (T_R = 450 msec).

3. (a) 900/100 intensities:

Spleen:

$$I = N(1 - e^{-900/900})e^{-200/100}$$

$$= N(1 - 0.368)(0.135) = 0.09\ N$$

Adjacent tissue:

$$I = N(1 - e^{-900/225})e^{-200/50}$$

$$= N(1 - 0.02)0.02 = .02\ N$$

Ratio: $0.09/0.02 = 4.5$.

(b) 900/50 intensities:

Spleen:

$$I = N(1 - e^{-900/900})e^{-100/100}$$

$$= N(1 - 0.368)0.368 = 0.23\ N$$

Adjacent tissue:

$$I = N(1 - e^{-900/225})e^{-100/50}$$

$$= N(1 - 0.02)0.135\ N = 0.13\ N$$

Ratio: $0.23/0.13 = 1.8$.

900/50. Although the sequence 900/100 produces a higher intensity ratio, the proton density of spleen (0.09 N) and adjacent tissue (0.02 N) detected by this sequence is extremely small. As a consequence, the images would be extremely noisy. The noise itself would interfere with the distinction between the two tissues. Contrast alone is not a sufficient criterion for the selection of pulse sequences, rather it is the contrast: noise ratio. This subject will be considered in the next textbook.

4. (a) 5000/500 intensities:

Compartment (1):

$$I = N(1 - e^{-5000/1000})e^{-100/100}$$

$$= N(1)(0.368) = 0.368\ N$$

Compartment (2):

$$I = N(1 - e^{-5000/500})e^{-100/50}$$

$$= N(1)(0.135) = 0.135\ N$$

Ratio: $0.368/0.135 = 2.73$.

(b) 1000/50 intensities:

Compartment (1):

$$I = N(1 - e^{-1000/1000})e^{-100/100}$$

$$= N(0.632)0.368 = 0.23\ N$$

Compartment (2):

$$I = N(1 - e^{1000/500})e^{-100/50}$$

$$= N(0.865)0.135 = 0.12\ N$$

Ratio: $0.23/0.12 = 1.92$.

The 1000/50 sequence would be the sequence of choice because the intensity ratio is very large (even though not as large as that for the 5000/50 sequence), the intensities from the compartments are large, and *only* ⅕ *the time is required to obtain the imaging data.*

5. The 1000/50 sequence would be the one of choice because the 1000/200 sequence would result in extremely noisy images with very little proton intensity contributed by either compartment 1: $(e^{-400/100} \sim 0\ N)$ or compartment 2: $(e^{-400/50} \sim 0\ N)$.

Set B

1. F	26. F
2. T	27. T
3. F	28. T
4. T	29. F
5. F	30. F
6. F	31. T
7. F	32. T
8. F	33. T
9. F	34. F
10. T	35. T
11. T	36. T
12. F	37. T
13. T	38. F
14. T	39. T
15. T	40. F
16. F	41. F
17. F	42. F
18. T	43. T
19. T	44. T
20. F	45. T
21. T	46. T
22. T	47. T
23. T	48. T
24. T	49. F
25. T	50. T

Suggested Reading List

Bradley WG, Newton TH, Crooks LE. Physical principles of nuclear magnetic resonance. In Newton TH, Potts DG, eds., *Advanced imaging techniques,* Modern Neuroradiology 2, San Anselmo, California: Clavadel Press, 1983; 15–61.

This compact, well-written overview of the basic physics of NMR imaging gently introduces the reader to the proton as a magnetic dipole having quantized energy states. Magnetization, phase coherence, relaxation, instrumentation, and a comparison of pulse sequences and imaging techniques are presented.

Brant-Zawadzki M, Norman D, eds. Magnetic resonance imaging of the central nervous system. New York: Raven Press, 1987.

This book contains well-written chapters on the basic physics and technical aspects of proton magnetic resonance imaging followed by chapters on the appearance of T_1 and T_2 weighted proton images of the normal CNS and disorders of the CNS.

Daniels DL, Haughton VM, Naidich TP, eds. Cranial and spinal magnetic resonance imaging: an atlas and guide. New York: Raven Press, 1987.

This book illustrates the variation with pulse parameters of spin-echo MRIs of normal and diseased CNS. It provides detailed comparisons of these images with anatomic dissections, cryomicrotomic sections, and histologic preparations.

Higgins CB, Hricak H, eds. Magnetic resonance imaging of the body. New York: Raven Press, 1987.

This book contains valuable descriptions of the basic physical principals, technical aspects, and safety and economic considerations in proton magnetic resonance imaging and a comprehensive survey of clinical proton imaging of the body.

Middleton WD, Lawson TL, eds. Anatomy and MRI of the joints: a multiplanar atlas. New York: Raven Press, 1989.

This book compares T_1 weighted proton images of the joints with cryomicrotomic serial sections obtained from cadavers.

Mink JH, Reicher MA, Crues JV III, eds. Magnetic resonance imaging of the knee. New York: Raven Press, 1987.

Following a technical overview of magnetic resonance imaging, this book provides a detailed comparison of T_1 and T_2 weighted spin-echo proton magnetic resonance images of the normal knee and disorders of the knee with drawings of the knee and with photographs of cryomicrotomic sections of the knees of cadavers.

Pykett IL. NMR imaging in medicine. *Sci Am* 1982 246: 78–88.

This is a notable, early, but still relevant attempt to explain the physics of NMR imaging.

Stark DD, Bradley WG, eds. Magnetic resonance imaging. St. Louis: C.V. Mosby Co., 1988.

This is a weighty comprehensive tome of approximately 1500 pages containing contributions from 42 authors in 47 chapters and a glossary of NMR terms. It covers the basic physics, technical aspects, and safety and economic considerations in magnetic resonance imaging followed by a detailed discussion of clinical imaging of the CNS and body.

Wehrli FW, Shaw D, Kneeland JB, eds. Biomedical magnetic resonance imaging: principles, methodology, and applications. New York: VCH Publishers, Inc., 1988.

This also is an advanced comprehensive text of approximately 600 pages in 13 chapters by 19 authors. Although the coverage of clinical proton imaging is comprehensive, the emphasis in this book is on the basics of MRI.

Young SW. Magnetic resonance imaging: basic principles, 2nd ed., New York: Raven Press, 1988.

An overview of the basic physics of proton NMR imaging is followed by a discussion of the clinical applications of proton NMR using images obtained with different pulse sequences, fields of view, and resolution. A glossary of MRI terms and an atlas of normal MRI anatomy are included along with a short discussion of NMR spectroscopy, imaging other nuclei (^{23}Na, ^{13}C, ^{19}F), hazards and site planning, and MRI economics.

Subject Index

A

Alternating current, *see* Voltage
Angular momentum, 45–47
Attenuated contrast
T_1 (weighted), 77–78
T_2 (weighted), 81–82
and echo evolution time, 81–82
and head images, 97–104
and image intensities, 83–84
and repetition time, 77–78
and T_1 and T_2 changes, 83–84

B

Bird cage coils, 42
Body coils, 41–42
Brain
lipid protons, 85–86
spin echo images, 97–104

C

Cerebrospinal fluid, 97, 100–102
Coil shape, 35, 39, 41
and magnetic fields, 35
Computer component, 42–43
Contrast effects
and echo evolution time, 81–82,
83–84, 97–104
head images, 97–104
and repetition time, 77–79, 83–84,
97–104
signal intensity role, 82
Convoluted (composite) free induction
decay, 89
"Cool" spin system, 70

D

Deconvoluted free induction decay, 89,
91–93
"Dephasing"
and shape of slice selection gradients,
93
by field inhomogeneities, 61–63, 79
by fluctuating tissue magnetization,
64–65, 66–68
irreversible, 68, 80
lipid magnetization, 85
nonrandom processes, 63
random processes, 68, 80
water protons, 64–68

E

Echo evolution time (T_E)
contrast effects, 81–82, 83–84, 97–104
dephasing recovery, 79–80
head images, 97–104
and π pulses, 79–80
Electrical current, 1–3, 17–19, 34–36,
37–38
Electromagnets, 36–37
Electromotive force, *see* Voltage
Exponential processes, 71–73, 78, 82

F

Faraday's Law, 7
Fats, *see* Lipid protons
Ferrite, 33–34
"Flickering clusters," 70
Flip angle, *see* Pulse angle
Fourier transformation, 93
Free induction decay, 61–63, 87–95
Free precession, 52, 56–57, 61

118 SUBJECT INDEX

Frequency
    encoding, 19–20, 26, 87–94
    in image construction, 87–95
    monitoring, 17–19
    quantitative considerations, 15–17
    shift by static field gradients, 19–20,
        87–94
Fringe fields, 34–36

G
Gadolinium
    diethylenetriaminepentaacetic acid,
        104
Gauss, 5
GdDTPA, 104
"Ghosts," 103
Glioblastoma, 102–103
Gradient coils
    amplifier rise time, 39
    configurations, 39
    linear gradient creation, 39
Gradient reversal, 93
Gray matter, 98, 100

H
"Hard" pulses, 55
Head images, 97–104
Heat, 69–71
Hertz, 8
Homogeneous magnetic field
    definition, 31–33
    and phase coherence, 61–64
"Hot" spin system, 70

I
Image intensity, *see* Signal intensity
Imaging time, 75–86
Intensity of signal, *see* Signal intensity
Intramolecular dipolar fields, 65
Intrinsic T_2 value, 80
Iron core electromagnets, 36–37

L
Larmor equation, 8, 46
Larmor frequency, *see* Resonance
    frequency
Lipid protons
    in brain, 85
    and relaxation processes, 85–86
Liquid helium, 38
Liquid nitrogen, 38
Loop configuration, wire, 34–36
Low-field magnets, 33

M
Macromolecules
    spin-lattice relaxation effect, 70
    water proton interactions, 66–67, 70
Magnet shimming, 40
Magnetic field; *see* Oscillating magnetic
    field; Static magnetic field
Magnetic Field Gradients
    definition, 11–12
    and frequency encoding, 19–20,
        25–28, 87–94
    and phase encoding, 22–25, 25–28,
        87–94
    and slice selection, 12–13
Magnetic moment
    macromolecules, 66–68
    and proton spin concept, 45–47
    and three-dimensional model, 47–48
    water, fluctuation, 64–68
Magnetism, 17–19
Magnetization
    basic principles, 3–5
    precession, 56–57, 61–63
    and relaxation, 59–61, 68–71
    rotation of, 54–56
    three-dimensional model, 45–49, 52–54
    two-dimensional model, 45
    tissue protons, 4–7
Magnetogyric ratio
    definition, 8, 46
    protons, 62
Megahertz, 8
Minicomputer, 43
Motion effects, 103

N
Niobium/titanium, 37–38

O
Orienting field, *see* Static magnetic field
Oscillating current, 6–7
Oscillating magnetic field (B_1)
    properties, 50–51
    proton signal creation, 50–54
    and pulse angles, 54–56
    quantitative concepts, 17–19
Oscillation frequency, *see* Resonance
    frequency
Out of phase concept, *see* Phase shift

P
Passive shimming, 40
Permanent magnets
    field shape, 31–33
    low-field MRI, 33

SUBJECT INDEX   119

Phase
   in image construction, pixels, 87–95
   and three-dimensional model, 47–49
   and two-dimensional model, 21–25
Phase coherence
   creation of, 52–54
   field inhomogeneity destruction of,
      61–64
   and spin-spin relaxation, 63
Phase shift
   basic concept, 21–22
   by static field gradients, 21–25, 87–94
   and voltage, 21–22
   water proton, macromolecule effect,
      67
Pixels, 87–95
Precession; *see also* Free precession
   concept of, 46–47
   and signal generation, 56–57
   xy plane, 56–57
Proteins
   spin-lattice relaxation effect, 70
   water proton interactions, 66–67, 70
Proton density
   definition, 1, 13, 25
   head imaging, values, 97, 100–102
   image construction, pixels, 87–95
   pixel assignment, 90
   and signal intensity, 77–79, 83–84
Protons
   magnetization of, 4–7, 45–46
   resonance frequency, 7–8, 46
   three-dimensional model for
      precession, 45–48
Pulse angle
   and oscillating magnetic field, 54–56
   radians, 55

R

Radians, 55
Radiofrequency coils, 41–42
Radiofrequency field, 50–54
Random fluctuating fields, 68
Random phase, 49
Receiver coil, 10
Reciprocity principle, 18–19, 50
Relaxation processes, 59–61 (*see also*
   Spin-lattice relaxation; Spin-spin
   relaxation)
Repetition time (T_R)
   contrast effects, head, 97–104
   contrast effects, signal intensity, 77–78
   and spin-lattice relaxation, 75–77
Resistive electromagnets, 36–37
Resonance frequency
   concept, 8–12
   and oscillating field, 10–12, 52–53
   and precession, 46
   and static magnetic field, 7–8

Reversed gradient, 93
Right hand rule, 18–19

S

Scalp, 98, 100–102
Shielded solenoids, 36
Shimming, 40
Signal frequency, *see* Frequency
Signal intensity, 75–86
   echo evolution time effect, 81–82,
      83–84, 97–104
   head images, 97–104
   image construction, pixels, 90–92
   and repetition time, 77–79, 83–84,
      97–104
Signal phase, *see* Phase
"Soft" pulses, 55
Solenoid configuration, 34–36
Spin, classical concept, 45–47
Spin echo
   definition, 79–80
   dephasing recovery, 79–81
   head images, 97–104
Spin-lattice relaxation (T_1)
   contrast influence, 75–86, 97–104
   definition, 63, 68–70
   exponential processes, 71–73
   general aspects, 68–71
   head images, 97–104
   imaging time/intensity influence,
      75–86, 97–104
   and lipids, 85–86
   versus spin-spin relaxation, 71–73
   time dependencies, 71–73
   water protons, 70
Spin-spin relaxation (T_2)
   contrast influence, 75–86, 97–104
   definition, 63
   exponential processes, 71–73
   head images, 97–104
   imaging time/intensity influence, 75–86
   intrinsic values, 80
   macromolecule effect, 66–68
   versus spin-lattice relaxation, 71–73
   time dependencies, 71–73
Static magnetic field
   and electric currents, 3, 17–19, 34–36,
      39
   in homogeneities, 31–33, 61–63, 79–80
   and phase shift, 22–25
   and the proton, 1–2, 45–47
   quantitative concepts, 17–19
   and resonance frequency, 7–8, 19–20
   shimming, 40
Superconducting magnet
   advantages and disadvantages, 38
   characteristics, 37–38
   fringe fields, 34–36
Surface coils, 41–42

T

Tesla, 5
Three-dimensional oscillation, 45–58
Time dependencies, relaxation, 71–73
"Time to echo," 80–82
Tissue protons, 4–7
Transceiver, 10
Transmitter coil, 10
True T_2 value, 80–86
2D Fourier transformation, 93

V

Vectors
  addition, 25, 49, 51
  magnetic moment, 47–48
  and phase shift, 24–25
  projections, 15–17, 47–48
Voltage
  and oscillating magnetic moment,
    17–19, 56–57, 62
  and phase shift, 21–22

W

Water "lattice," 69
Water protons
  intramolecular dipolar fields, 65

macromolecules effect, dephasing,
    66–68
  magnetic moment oscillation, 64–66
  versus lipid protons, 85–86
Weak pulses, 55
Weighted contrast, *see* Attenuated
    contrast
White matter, 98, 100

X

X coordinate
  proton density mapping, 25–28
XY plane
  frequency and phase, 15–29
  magnetization precessing, 56–57
  phase coherence creation, 52–54
  proton density mapping, 15–29

Y

Y coordinate
  proton density mapping, 25–28

Z

Z coordinate
  proton density mapping, 25–28
  in three-dimensional model, 47–48